"This book provides information and advice essential to helping bariatric patients succeed at weight loss surgery."
~ Emily Neller, M.A., therapist for bariatric patients

"Weight loss doesn't have to change just within our stomach, but within our minds, too. Getting to the root of the problem is an essential part of success and *Eat it Up!* is needed to address those issues."
~ Amy Williams, Bariatric Patient Advocate, Jones Hill & Blaney, MDs Augusta, GA

"This book is a much-needed resource to help weight loss surgery patients deal with the emotional issues that crop up after surgery."
~ Bryn Hamilton, RD, LD and LapBand patient

"A great tool to assist patients in the journey of bariatric surgery."
~ Jo Anne Robinson, bariatric patient

"It is really important to have a book for bariatric patients that focuses on more than just the ins and outs of the surgery itself, but the life we are left with after the fact."
~ Rebecca Poole-Ward, bariatric patient; medical student

"I have to tell you how much I ADORE your book. It should be a book club read staple for EVERY Support group. I am going to incorporate your book into a project. It is amazing."
~ Laura Preston, Bariatric Patient; Queen of the Blog
– http://www.mydailydetour.com

EAT IT UP!

The Complete Mind/Body/Spirit Guide to a
Full Life After Weight Loss Survey

CONNIE STAPLETON, PH.D.

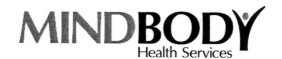

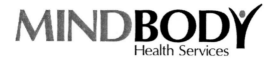

Published by Mind Body Health Services, Inc.

ISBN: 978-0692500637

Library of Congress Control Number: 2009928681

This book is printed on acid free paper.

Printed in the USA

DEDICATION

For every person who has known the pain of obesity and who is ready to live a full, balanced life, I offer you inspiration gained from others who have gone before you. With gratitude, I share their courage, strength and hope… may you *Eat It Up!*

ACKNOWLEDGEMENTS

This is my favorite page of the book! First and foremost, I share my love and gratitude for the gifts of tremendous love, patience, and encouragement from my husband of a quarter century who I admire, respect and treasure. Steve, you have shared with me a love and a partnership beyond anything I thought possible in this world. Thank you for taking on so much of the work in this venture and in all that we do! You are my hero, every day, time and time again.

Steven, my son, your generosity with time, technical support, advice and creativity led to this book, including the front and back covers, becoming a 3-D reality. I thank you for your willingness to teach and re-teach me things over and over again on the computer. You are an incredible man. I am excited about your life, am so grateful for you and am proud that you are my son!

Erin, my daughter and publicist, I very much appreciate the thankless work you have put into this project thus far and thank you in advance for the hundreds of hours of work you have ahead! Working with you is a dream come true and a privilege for me! You have no idea yet of the talents and gifts you possess, beautiful woman, but I look forward to watching you figure it out!

Kelsey, your love, encouragement and enthusiasm for my work provides fuel for my body and soul when I need refreshing. Thank you for shining your light so brightly on my life and in this world. I so very much appreciate your gentle nudges to keep my chin up and your energizing hugs every time I see you! Watching you touch the lives of so many makes my heart sing.

Mom, thank you for keeping me laughing, and for sharing your fascinating gift of wonder about life and your unique, wonderfully curious and creative nature. Your example of taking risks, following your dreams and sharing abundance with others live in me as an honor to your teachings. Thank you for sharing your life with my family.

Diane, my soul-sister, thank you for being my friend no matter what and for our love, always and forever. Susie, you are my angel on earth. I aspire to be more like you and am grateful for your love, your example of faith, and your incredible laughter. Sally, thank you for "getting me," for playing and for sharing Simon with me. Thank you too, for educating me from a first-hand perspective! Casa, you make me laugh more than anyone else in this world; thank you for that and for participating in all of my most important events. Wanda, thank you for checking on me and loving me every day. Boo, for a lifetime of friendship and encouragement, I thank you. DiDi, I love you and miss you always. Carol, your teaching, love and understanding mean more to me than you will ever know. Kathy, I miss you all the time and treasure every rare minute we get to share. Amanda, Megan, and Emily, how lucky I am to have gotten to add you to my life most recently! Thank you all for putting up with this parroting pirate! I really love and appreciate you. Bob, your sign has been a constant inspiration to me. You'll never know.

Karen Wall, I cannot imagine where my life would have gone (nor do I want to), if God had not put me in your path. There are no earthly words or feelings to describe my gratitude to you or my love for you. Thank you, thank you, thank you.

John Friel, you will never know the impact your work and books have had on my life. Thank you for teaching me - during the short time I got to work with you and ever since through your writing. Much gratitude to you.

Ginny Weissman, thank you for leading me into this world of authordom. You hold my hand from across the country! I can't tell you how grateful I am for your part in helping me turn my dreams into realities. Thank you for believing in this project and for following through with it. Paul Burt. Wow! Your knowledge and guidance are appreciated beyond measure. Thank you for your honesty and direct approach. Lauren Bryant, I am so grateful for your time, your talent and your willingness to help out! Thank you for your editing contribution to this project.

To the awesome group I work with at Trinity Bariatric Center, I thank you for the fun we have and the support you give me. Dr. Blaney, Dr, Chasen, Bryn, Cathie, Dana, Amy, Tosca, and Carla, thanks much! I also appreciate the surgeons and staff at the South Carolina Obesity Surgery Center. And to those at ObesityHelp.com who have given me so many awesome opportunities to write and speak – Kim, Cathy, Bo, Tammy, Jeremy, Jeannie and the rest - I treasure your encouragement and thank you from my heart.

To every patient I have had the privilege of working with, I thank you. Thank you for allowing me into your world and for trusting me with your feelings. I pray to be of service to you and to inspire you in the best ways I know how (i.e., however God guides me).

God – for your guidance and love, I thank you. I am so very grateful for the honor of sharing in the lives of so many great people and for the opportunities to work with others. Mostly, I appreciate the husband and children you are sharing with me. Help me to give back to others through my work in the ways that all of the people mentioned here have shared with me in helping me along my journey.

Table of Contents

Chapter 1

Fully Forward

Here are five things your bariatric surgeon didn't tell you:
- his mother's maiden name
- the street she grew up on
- the name of his first pet
- her husband's favorite teacher
- the fact that a significant percentage of weight loss surgery patients will regain a great deal of their weight in two to five years following surgery.

During the weeks and months leading to your surgery, you probably did more research than you did in all of your years of schooling combined. Do you recall reading anywhere about the number of people who regain some or all of their pre-surgery weight a year, or two years, or five years after surgery?

Even if you ran across such information, you likely breezed right over it, scarcely giving it a thought, knowing that you would not be one of *those* people! Like the young bride and bridegroom preparing for their wedding who are certain they will not be in the fifty percent of marriages that end in divorce, you proceeded with confidence, knowing you would be a successful weight loss patient.

My job, while encouraging and supporting your post-surgery efforts, is to also point out the not-so-fun facts. Couples who have been married for many years are aware of the effort it takes to have a successful marriage. They know it is not all fun and games. Those rings and that marriage license do not guarantee Happily Ever After. Neither do the stitches indicating that your bariatric surgery is complete, nor do the papers discharging you from the hospital guarantee Happily Ever After.

Wait! Don't close the book now and run away scared! I'm not trying to be a dooms-dayer who bursts your bubbles of happiness, excitement and anticipation. I'm on your side. Choosing to have bariatric surgery is one of the most important decisions you have ever made for yourself. I am here to encourage and support you. I can also supply you with additional knowledge and skills to help ensure your success. My goal is to bolster your confidence in staying the course, in keeping your weight off, and in finding a Happily Ever After that is real and far better than in any fairy tale.

Couples who have been happily married for years and years know that having a solid, happy marriage requires hard work. There are rough times and smooth times. Times you do things even though you don't feel like it, yet you do what needs to be done because it will benefit the relationship. At times you wonder what you have gotten yourself into, but because you made the decision to get married, you persist in keeping true to your vows. In the end, those who stick it out are proud of what they have accomplished. They are confident that the benefits of their marriage far outweigh the struggles.

So it is with life after bariatric surgery. You embarked on the journey, as you should, starry-eyed, unable to wait for The Big Day, and thrilled about the prospect of the honeymoon! You knew that "real life" would begin soon enough. And you were ready for that, too. Because now, like the young newlyweds who have finally found their life partner, you have what you are certain will lead to your lifelong happiness. Having weight loss surgery meant a way for you to really and truly lose weight, and to you, that has always meant that you would finally be happy. To be sure, there will be times you won't feel like following through with behavior that is good for you (exercise; refraining from dessert; completing food and exercise diaries.) You will do it, though, because you made a commitment. You also know these behaviors are essential for your long-term goals of sustained weight loss and happiness. There will be times when you wonder what you have gotten yourself into. You will then reaffirm your commitment to your health and happiness and persist in doing "the next right thing," whatever that is at the moment. In the end, like the couple who joyfully celebrates their 50th wedding anniversary, you will rejoice knowing you made the choice to have a healthy body, to live life fully and to *Eat It Up!*

That surgeon who failed to mention the patients who regain their weight did not mean to mislead you. He was likely thinking about "success" from the medical perspective, which to him, means that you will lose fifty percent of your excess weight. Your health will be improved and he will have what he desired: another medical success. (Well-meaning parents sometimes forget to mention the peaks and valleys of marriage as their youngsters wed because, whether the young couple stays together or not, the parents are likely to get what they wanted: grandchildren!) My purpose in writing this book is to guide you, from the day you have your surgery, through the ups and downs of daily life as a post-surgical patient, to successful long-term weight loss and a genuinely happy, balanced life. I want to educate and inspire you so you don't regain the weight you lose. I must, therefore, provide you with the realities of life after bariatric surgery.

I work on a daily basis directly with the bariatric population and see first-hand the emotional struggles clients go through in the days, weeks, months, and yes, the years following bariatric surgery. Sadly, I have seen the devastation people suffer by regaining pound after pound of weight that had been lost in the months immediately following surgery. I can help you prevent the regaining of weight. Of course, you are the one who has to make the decision to take the information I provide and practice it in your life on a daily basis. I have read most of the books on the market about pre- and post- weight loss surgery. I attended Harvard's annual International Conference on the Practical Treatment of Obesity. I have been through Harvard's Mind/Body training presented by Herbert Benson, MD, creator of "The Relaxation Response" and author of the book of the same title. I have done my homework. And I work in the field. In working with and listening to bariatric patients in my work, I help them understand what they know on a cognitive level: weight loss surgery is only the beginning of the happy, balanced life they are seeking. Regardless, each one hopes that the surgery will be The Answer and "Everything Else" will simply and magically fall into place after that. "Everything Else" includes:

- I will no longer have cravings for the foods I love.
- My car will automatically ignore all fast food drive-thrus.
- My habit of going to the refrigerator/cupboards every fifteen minutes will disappear.
- I will develop an intense love and desire for 60 to 90 minutes of daily exercise.
- I will refuse to take escalators when stairs are available; I will prefer to walk without the benefit of the moving sidewalk in the airport; and I will happily park as far away from the store as possible for the sheer pleasure of taking those extra steps.
- I will have foolproof resistance to the smorgasbord of food at family reunions, holidays and social gatherings.

Here is one of those realities mentioned earlier: bariatric surgery does primarily one thing. Bariatric surgery decreases the physical size of the area of your stomach that can hold food. That's it. Nothing less. Nothing more. (Okay, so depending on the type of procedure you have, the intestines may be rerouted, as well.) The point is, surgery does absolutely nothing to deal with the two things that are primarily responsible for the regaining of weight after bariatric surgery: your long-term eating and exercise habits and the cognitive and emotional issues related to those eating and exercise behaviors. The fact is, without addressing the cognitive, emotional and behavioral issues underlying obesity, weight loss surgery is actually a very expensive and invasive "diet." And like the other diets you have tried, it is doomed to fail unless you do the work suggested in this book.

That is why I wrote this book. I can help you with those things. The best-selling books on bariatric surgery on the market primarily address the decision-making process leading to surgery and the medical aspects of bariatric surgery. *Eat It Up!* guides you through the process of exploring the cognitive, emotional and behavioral components that ultimately determine if you will succeed in sustaining your weight loss or if you will have spent thousands of dollars on yet another failed diet. In addition, in *Eat It Up!* you are given exercises to do in each chapter that are geared to lead you to success. If you do them there is no reason you will not reach the weight goals you have set. Beyond that, you will experience the transition from a world that has been like an old television show experienced in only black and white to a life that is exploding in full, brilliant color! The difference is indescribable. The choice is yours.

If you think you don't need this information, then put the book down, but don't get rid of it. I believe there will be a time in the future when you will want and need this information. I recommend, in fact, that you read through the book once from start to finish. Then start again at the beginning and go through it slowly, working on the exercises you feel you need. Do this all the way through the book, in order. Then, over time, as you encounter situations in your daily life that you are struggling with, come back to this book, find the section related to a particular issue, and work through the exercises again. We all grow and change with time. The thoughts, feelings and ideas you have related to a particular issue will change as you change. The information in this book is here to provide assistance. It's yours to use or not. I hope you will choose to use it. Again and again.

Your Whole Self

I take a mind/body/spirit approach in my work, and in writing about your overall success following weight loss surgery. To me, this translates to permanent weight loss following surgery and finding the happiness you have been seeking. Since this book is designed to help you prevent weight regain, I will share what I know about that particular topic. However, I am going to go further than simply suggesting you put the right foods into your body and get sufficient exercise. I am going to address how your obesity and your weight loss surgery are intertwined with your whole self: body, mind, and spirit. I do this by focusing on six major areas of your life, or Centers of Balance, which include your Physical Center, your Cognitive Center, your Emotional Center, your Social Center, your Spiritual Center, and your Enterprise Center. I am positive that by choosing to follow the suggestions provided in this book, you will live out your Happily Ever After in your thinner, healthier body.

Your Centers of Balance: Your True Keys to Happiness

For so long, diet after diet, through weight loss and weight regain, you have clung to the notion that when you lost your excess weight, you would be happy. If that were the case, people would not regain their weight after a successful diet. Weight loss surgery patients that have gone before you would be living the blissfully happy lives they presumed being thinner would bring them. We all know that weight loss alone does not mean inevitable happiness.

The happiest, most functional people in our society live balanced lives. I describe a balanced life in terms of six Centers of Balance. The happy, functional people I speak of spend time in solitude or prayer and carry the benefits into their lives while still dealing with "the real world" (Spiritual Center). They put effort into keeping their thoughts and feelings in a moderate range. They are not ruled by rigid thoughts or out-of-control emotions, nor are they emotionally shut down or blunted (Cognitive Center and Emotional Center). They spend time with friends, but not at the expense of their families or other responsibilities (Social Center). They get both aerobic and anaerobic exercise on a regular basis and engage in physical activity, but don't take it to the extremes (Physical Center). They work, but don't overdo it. They give back to their communities through volunteer or service work, while taking care of themselves and their families or other responsibilities (Enterprise Center). My goal is to address your real-life issues related to life following bariatric surgery in the context of your Centers of Balance. The result: you will live the well-balanced life of one of the genuinely happy people in our world in your new, more physically healthy body, keeping your weight off throughout your lifetime.

In Chapter 2, you will take a journey into your past. We'll explore the reasons for obesity, including physiological and emotional components. Exercises guide you in taking an overall inventory of the factors leading to your obesity. You will determine the issues you need to work on to prevent the return of bad habits leading to weight regain as you move toward your healthier life.

In Chapter 3, you take stock of your spiritual beliefs and practices. Your Spiritual Center is the epicenter of your life. Being obese has interfered in your relationship with God, your relationship with yourself and your relationships with others. Obesity is a disease of isolation. Angry about being judged and ridiculed, you became isolated. Shame and embarrassment led to further isolation. Thought-provoking questions help you determine how your authentic self got lost in the process of becoming obese. You will choose how to use spiritual principles to guide you in the process of regaining your authentic self throughout your recovery from obesity.

Chapter 4 is the most difficult chapter in the book. You learn how your thoughts, feelings and behaviors are intertwined. Obesity weighed you down with negative messages about yourself, about what you could do and about what you were worth. Negative thoughts and feelings kept you imprisoned, as did your obesity. Here you will address issues from the past so that you can work through them and move beyond them. You will develop positive thinking habits, which will impact your feelings and your behaviors in healthy ways. You'll learn tools to help prevent sabotage by self and others. You'll set goals for developing healthy behaviors, you'll accept responsibility for the choices you make, and you'll move toward health and happiness.

In Chapter 5, I tackle the world of physical exercise and activity. You can vent and whine and complain if you hate exercise. You can rejoice if you love it and can't wait to get to it. No matter what, you will partake in it as there is no way to avoid exercise if you want to lose weight and keep it off. You will choose how to make exercise fun, and if that concept doesn't stand a chance of working for you, then you can use other options presented in the chapter to motivate yourself to get out there and sweat.

Chapter 6 focuses on the social aspects of your life and the dramatic changes that take place in your social life after surgery. The shame associated with being obese led to social and emotional isolation as well as spiritual isolation. After you lose weight, your self-esteem improves, and your interactions with others change accordingly. These changes are received well by some but not so happily by others. Learning to be assertive and to set healthy boundaries will further enhance your sense of self-worth. Inviting your family and loved ones to join you as you change and grow will make your transition to healthy living smoother for you and those you love.

Chapter 7 focuses on your Enterprise Center. Your Enterprise Center includes what you do for work, how you enhance your mind, what your hobbies are, how you handle your finances, and the ways you contribute to society. Being obese stole opportunities from you in each of these areas. To rebalance this Center, you will identify messages you were given and that you continue to give yourself regarding your worth and ability. Expanding your life leads to better self esteem, healthier thoughts and improved feelings, which translates to overall improved health, happiness and sustained weight loss.

Chapter 8 is called The Road Infrequently Traveled. Unlike diets from yesteryear that you "went on" and "came off of," the behaviors you choose following bariatric surgery are lifelong, permanent changes. Perseverance is the road infrequently traveled by post-surgical patients. As adults, we are responsible for making positive choices regarding our health. If you use the skills taught throughout this book every day, one day and one choice at a time, referring to this guidebook often and completing the exercises, you will find success!

Fully Forward

Congratulations. You have an idea of what lies ahead: hard work, tears and painful feelings. I'll bet you can hardly wait to get started! Take heart. The best truly is yet to come. Move fully forward through the rough patches because on the other side, you will be living a fully healthy, happy and balanced life. *Eat It Up!*

Chapter 2

Your Cup Runneth Dry:
Obesity and Your Centers of Balance

When did you decide you wanted to be fat? You're probably wondering if I've lost my mind asking a question like that. The truth is, I have never had a client tell me he or she decided, chose, or wanted to be fat – ever. So, how did you end up becoming obese?

As you already know, various factors account for obesity. When you first saw your bariatric surgeon, what did you tell her about the reasons for your obesity? Did you say you that were fat from day one? That you didn't gain weight until you became pregnant? That your entire family consisted of obese people and that genetically, you didn't stand a chance? That you were a size two until you got married, but then you steadily gained weight over the years? That your thyroid was under functioning? Any of these statements may be true.

But what did you *not* tell your surgeon about your weight history? That your mom, who was obese herself (or, conversely, as thin as a rail) commented on every morsel of food you put into your mouth and that you eventually became just as obsessed with every morsel of food you ate? That you started gaining weight in the fifth grade because you didn't want to attract physical attention to yourself after your uncle touched you where he shouldn't have? That your home was a battleground where your parents were constantly at war with one another, and your only source of comfort was food? That you were deprived of candy or any form of dessert because your father didn't want any fat daughters? That you were the only male in the family who was made fun of because you were clumsy and not good at sports, so you found solace in food? That you became chunky so you no longer had to try out for sports, which you didn't like in the first place?

Which is the truth? The information you gave your surgeon, the information you left out, or both? The things you did tell the surgeon are undoubtedly part of your true history. Some or all of the factors contributing to your obesity may be outside of your awareness. What you believe, or are aware of, about the cause of your obesity will likely change as you lose weight. If that sounds odd, ask people you know who have already had bariatric surgery and have lost 50 or 70 or 100 pounds. They are likely to chuckle, thinking about how their thoughts related to their own obesity have changed since having surgery and losing weight.

Michelle, a 30-year-old second grade teacher who lost 110 pounds in the year following her surgery, blushed when she told me, "I always told people I was a fat kid because I didn't like to play outside. As an adult, I used the excuse of not liking exercise as the reason I remained heavy. Now I am able to recognize, and to say out loud, that the real reason I stayed in the house and ate when I was young was because the boys in the neighborhood called me fat. They still trapped me on the playground and fondled me, fat and all. I was humiliated, scared, and angry. I never talked to anyone about it until now."

Marcus, a 42-year-old sales manager said, "Before I lost 200 pounds, I blamed my mom for my obesity because she is such a good cook. Now I can admit that I used her cooking as an excuse for my weight. I'm 42 years old and have lived on my own for 21 years. It can't be Mom's fault I remained obese until last year."

As people lose weight following bariatric surgery, they gain insight into their prior eating behaviors and the emotional reasons underneath their obesity.

The Physiological Facts
Genetics
- Fran accurately told her surgeon, "Every woman on my mother's side of the family is heavy." Fran has a genetic component to her obesity. Medical facts indicate that genetics account for approximately one-third of the reason a person is overweight or obese. Two-thirds of your obesity is related to factors other than genetics.

Thyroid Problems
- The thyroid has been a biological scapegoat for causing obesity. Unfairly and inaccurately so. The truth is that a malfunctioning thyroid is only minimally responsible for a person's weight change, whether that is weight gain or weight loss.

Medication
- If you want to blame something and sound credible doing so, blame your medications. A number of medications do result in weight gain. Certain prescription drugs used to treat mood disorders, seizures, migraines, diabetes, and even high blood pressure can cause weight gain. Some steroids, hormone replacement therapy, and oral contraceptives can also result in unwanted pounds.

Disease
- Some illnesses, including hormone problems, depression and some rare diseases of the brain can lead to obesity.

More often, there are other, more powerful reasons for a person's obesity. Physiological factors are only part of the story. The majority of the story behind a person's obesity is about unhealthy food choices, the lack of physical activity and exercise, negative emotions, and psychological issues.

The E Factors
One part genetics plus several parts environmental conditioning and emotional escape equals one hundred percent obesity.

Environment

Dorothy Law Nolte, Ph.D. wrote a painfully true, insightful poem entitled ***Children Learn What They Live***. Undeniably, children learn what they live in a home where one or more of the parents is obese. In fact, (sorry, moms) the number one determinant of childhood obesity is maternal obesity. Obese parents teach their children poor eating choices and habits. And so begins another generation of obese people.

Fran, the woman who told her surgeon that all of her female relatives are overweight, does very likely have a genetic marker for obesity. Yet the fact that all of the women in her family are overweight is due, in part, to their cooking and eating habits. Like other diseases, obesity is a combination of nature and nurture.

Emotions

Emotionally laden issues underlie a person's obesity. In his pre-surgical interview, Thomas, age 52, recounted the shame he felt every year when it was time to go back-to-school shopping. He was the only kid in the family who had to get "Husky" jeans. His siblings teased him. The worse he felt, the more he ate and the more weight he gained. He buried his shame beneath his fat.

After losing 160 pounds, Felicia tearfully shared this: "I hated the way kids stared at me when I was in school. Even when I became an adult, before I had the surgery, little kids still stared at me and called me 'Fatty.' I felt sad and angry and just wanted to hide when this happened, but God knows that hiding was impossible at 330 pounds." Felicia's obesity, as a child and adult, caused her great emotional pain.

The emotional heartache associated with obesity is as painful as the knee and joint pain associated with carrying 100 excess pounds. The emotional heartache hurts as badly as the back and leg and lung pain that an obese person experiences when climbing a flight of stairs. The emotional pain feeds on itself. The shame, embarrassment, anger, and fear associated with being overweight fuels the low self-worth experienced by obese people. Their low self-esteem emerges as negative self-talk, self-destructive behavior, and self-punishment, which leads to intensified feelings of hurt, sadness, shame, and rage. It is a cycle that turns continually, like a paddlewheel beneath a waterfall, and like the water rushing toward the fall, the pain never seems to end.

Your Life as a Cup

Rhonda, an intelligent, insightful woman in her late 50s, shared her reasons for deciding to have weight loss surgery. "My mother, on her death bed, told me that when I was born into this world, her mother, my grandmother, said I was a cup. My mother thought her mother was loony, yet gingerly asked what she meant. Grandma said that like every other child born into this world, I was born a full cup, a fully 'authentic person.' I was full of all of the 'good stuff' I would need to be happy in this world. I was full of love and kindness, joy and self-esteem, wonder and delight, compassion and generosity, faith and wisdom. My parents' job, Grandma said, was to not spill a single drop from my cup."

Rhonda's eyes shone as she shared her mother's tale. "My mother then apologized to me for spilling my cup when I was a child. What I realized," she went on, after wiping a tear, "is that as I was raised, more and more of my cup was spilled - some by my parents and some by mean kids at school - and then the worst thing of all happened. I started dumping it out myself. I have been nearly empty for a long time. It's like being spiritually bankrupt. The more that the 'good stuff' got poured out, the more I ate, trying to fill the cup back up. I got fat. I was no longer the person I was born into this world to be. Mom reminded me before she died that my 'authentic self' is still inside of me, a person created by God with a special purpose. She said she hoped I would try to find that person again."

"That's why I decided to have bariatric surgery," Rhonda continued. "I wanted to find my authentic self. I wanted to get rid of the fat and find healthy ways to fill my cup again and be who I was meant to be. I've lost 85 pounds so far and am learning how criticism and teasing spilled the 'good stuff' from my cup, as did witnessing the animosity between my parents. When I got older, I hated myself and spilled even more by getting in and out of abusive relationships, dropping out of college three times and losing scholarships, and by putting on more and more weight. I was punishing myself. Now, as I am learning to fill my cup back up in healthy ways, I'm starting to like myself. I can see that I have unique gifts and talents, and I am excited about finishing my degree and starting to teach. I will finally be living the life I was meant to live. I am becoming my authentic self."

The Empty, Unbalanced Cup of Obesity

Every day I work with wonderful human beings who have unique talents and gifts, whose Cups were spilled in a variety of ways during childhood. Their authentic selves became hidden beneath layers of fat. Their lives became unbalanced as each individual Center of Balance was knocked off course. As a person's Cup is spilled, their Centers of Balance are tilted. The results are the same: the person begins to look outside himself to fix the emptiness within. The obese person chooses food. More and more food is needed because it never takes the pain completely away, no matter how much is eaten. The authentic person is hidden. Hidden behind the food and hidden behind the fat.

An Unbalanced Spiritual Center

Once an adult, the now-obese person continues the unhealthy behaviors they learned in their youth. Food was an emotional comfort during difficult times then; it remains so in their adult life. Food was, and is, a way to hide from pain; a chance to experience sweetness in the bitterness of life. Their Spiritual Center, their connection to God, the world, and their authentic self becomes damaged. Their self-esteem erodes and increasing weight fills the void. As their Spiritual Center disintegrates, their authentic self shrinks. More and more weight. Less and less self-worth. All of their Centers of Balance are negatively impacted. When the Spiritual Center is tipped, all of the centers become off balance. It's like a mobile with zoo animals hanging over a baby's crib that gets bumped and all of the animals on the mobile start movin' and shakin'.

Bariatric surgery helps get rid of the fat but it cannot heal what is hidden beneath it. As fat melts away following bariatric surgery, long-buried thoughts and feelings of emptiness, sadness, shame, frustration, and anger surface. The disquieting thoughts and feelings are kept at bay by the excitement and attention generated by the rapid weight loss, the smaller clothes, and the new look. However, once the hype generated by the decreasing number on the scale simmers down and life settles into a new routine, up rise those same old miserable thoughts and feelings. If they are not acknowledged and the issues related to them are not addressed, food (or a substitute substance or negative behavior) is again used in an attempt to squelch the fire of feelings that rages internally. These negative thoughts and feelings and the resultant negative behaviors are the main reasons people regain their weight following bariatric surgery.

Unbalanced Cognitive and Emotional Centers

When it gets off kilter, the Cognitive Center of Balance can wreak havoc in other areas of life. Thoughts affect feelings and behavior.

"The hardest part for me," admitted Kathy, a 29-year-old accountant who dropped 40 pounds in the four months following her surgery, "is the way I keep thinking so negatively about myself. I mean, I'm proud of myself for making the decision to have the surgery and for doing what I am supposed to be doing every day. But I keep referring to myself as 'fat' and thinking I can't do this or that because I'm used to thinking that way."

Kathy has found articles on bariatric Web sites that address the importance of thinking positive thoughts about self in all dimensions of life. "As I get rid of the 'stinkin thinkin' habits of the old days and incorporate more optimistic thoughts, I feel better and am willing to take healthy risks in my life," Kathy said. "The results have been great. I like myself better and that seems to be contagious. I even have a third date with a great guy tonight!"

Unlike Kathy, who has taken positive steps toward becoming reacquainted with her authentic self, hundreds of thousands of overweight and obese people choose to stop living and merely exist. Some hope against hope that a new miracle diet will "work" and they will someday lose weight. Others relinquish hope, resigning themselves to a way of life that can accurately be described as a slow form of suicide. Their Centers of Balance are off their axes and their Cups remain drained.

Obese people opt for life on the roller coaster of losing and regaining weight. Emotionally, they experience the highs and lows accompanying their fluctuations in weight. Their behavior toward others is correspondingly inconsistent. Family members and loved ones are victims of their emotional swings. Children learn the dysfunctional responses associated with life in an imbalanced emotional environment.

Mary, a 41-year-old divorced mother of three, recalled her ex-husband telling her he could no longer endure the intensity of her mood swings related to weight. If a pair of pants was too tight Mary embarked on a tirade of negativity, and no one in the house was spared.

The purchase of a new outfit in "the right size" resulted in a celebration with a family outing to the movies. "No one ever knew what to expect," Mary sighed. Having lost 75 pounds since her weight loss surgery, she is now learning to modulate her behavior, regardless of her feelings. "I realize that my authentic self can respond appropriately in (almost) any situation. My kids seemed uncertain around me for a while because they were used to me being all over the place emotionally, but they are starting to trust that I will 'behave' myself, even if I feel uncomfortable in clothes that seem too tight."

An Unbalanced Physical Center

Physical activity all but halts for the obese person because of pain from a variety of body parts with even minimal physical exertion. "I missed my buddies," Rob said, although he admits he was reluctant to get together with the guys when he was obese. "I couldn't go hunting or fishing any more because of my weight. I couldn't keep up on the golf course. I just quit fitting in." After losing 80 pounds following his surgery, Rob joked, "I feel like a country song played backward... I have my wife back, my buddies back, and my life back!"

Linda's weight became so much a burden that "my young kids were left to play by themselves most of the time," she said. "Attending the older children's extracurricular activities decreased because it took so much effort to get off the couch."

Playing tennis, going on picnics, walking by the lake, and dancing become painful memories for the obese person when the Physical Center of Balance tips.

An Unbalanced Social Center

Countless clients report that before surgery, food was literally the center of their worlds. Male and female obese persons lack the energy, and eventually the desire, to engage with others. Their Social Centers slip. Relationships with loved ones often take second place to finding solace in the world of buffets, trips to the grocery store, or chips and a book.

"Rachel Ray, Emeril Lagasse, and any show on the Food Network took priority over time spent with my children," Kristine admitted. "Since losing weight, my kids tease me and ask me if I'm ever going to watch TV again. I'm too busy living to sit and watch television."

Intimacy between couples dwindles as increasing weight becomes a barrier. Michelle lamented, "I thought of myself as being physically repulsive. Sexual advances by my beloved husband would ignite the fire of self-loathing." As weight increases, physical contact diminishes, and sexual contact extinguishes.

Friendships also suffer for the obese person. Margaret said, "I became too self-conscious to be around other women. I preferred to remain alone in order to avoid any sort of scrutiny. I don't know if the scrutiny was real or imagined, but I stayed home most of the time before my surgery. It feels so good to go out into the world again!"

An Unbalanced Enterprise Center

"I kept going to work because I had to," Maureen recalled, 17 months and 120 pounds lighter after her surgery. "If I hadn't needed money (which I used primarily to afford my drive-thru restaurant habit), I would have quit my job like I quit everything else in my life. Since having surgery, I feel so alive again, actively participating in the Big Sisters program and taking my grandmother out for coffee."

Like people with drug and alcohol addictions or other behavioral addictions, obese people typically maintain their jobs until they are forced to quit or until they get fired. Other Enterprise Center activities, however, are among the first to go, as carrying excessive weight is emotionally and physically exhausting. Duane, a single 26-year-old male who is 95 pounds lighter seven months post-surgery, shared his enthusiasm for returning to the activities that "made my life my life." He resumed his participation as chairman of the local intramural basketball league, rejoined the Optimist Club, and plans to coach the high school debate team.

The Dumping and Refilling of Your Cup

The good news, in case your spirits are withering as you read this, is that by having bariatric surgery, you have taken a major step toward refilling your cup. Serious choices about if and how you choose to continue to refill your cup await you. The prize for doing so is finding your authentic self, who has hidden dormant inside you for a long, long time. Before the tools for helping you refill your cup are disclosed, we need to look more carefully at how it was dumped in the first place.

The Spilling of the Cup

Before you read this section, let me make a few extremely important points:

- I am not implying that your cup is completely empty. All people have their cups dumped at one time or another – that's what happens in life.
- The extent to which your cup has been dumped depends on the experiences you had as a child, how others have treated you in your adult life, and how you have treated yourself as an adult.
- I am not saying that your parents were, or are, bad parents.
- I am not asking you to blame anyone for your obesity. (I will discuss the difference between blame and accountability in a later chapter.)

Please read this section with a very open mind, and re-read it every six months or so from now on. You will be amazed at how your thoughts and feelings change over time as you continue to lose weight.

Imbalance Resulting from Neglect

When I talk with clients about how their cups were spilled, they often become quiet and distant. Very often people get defensive, as did Sherry. "I don't really understand why you think we have to discuss my childhood," she said. "My childhood is not related to my obesity. I had a very good childhood and very good parents. I didn't even gain weight until I was older and out of their house."

I assured Sherry that I believed she had positive experiences during her childhood, and that I was certain her parents were good people who loved her a great deal. But I urged her to share information about her childhood to see if there was any connection (even a slight one) between her obesity and her childhood experiences. She reluctantly agreed.

Sherry's mother was diagnosed with breast cancer when Sherry was 10 years old. Sherry had three younger siblings. Her mother's cancer metastasized, and she was sick at times over the next six years before passing away. During the years her mother was ill, Sherry assumed responsibility for her younger sisters. Their father was busy taking care of his wife and maintaining a job to support the family. Sherry said her parents were never critical of her, nor was there any sort of abuse.

Sherry needed help understanding that abuse is not the only thing that contributes to the loss of our authentic self. Although she had loving parents who were supportive of their children, Sherry's parents were focused on her Mother's physical care. The majority of Sherry's father's attention went to his wife and making sure the children had the physical necessities they needed. Sherry's mother, who did as much as she could for the family, was often too ill to be emotionally or physically available for the children.

Sometimes neglect occurs because of circumstances beyond anyone's control. In Sherry's family, no one had done anything "bad" or "wrong." The reality remained, however, that neither Sherry nor her siblings got the sufficient amount of emotional attention needed by children to mature in optimally healthy emotional ways. Sherry, in particular, being the oldest, took on overwhelming responsibilities for a child. She was not cognitively or emotionally equipped to deal with the chronic illness of one parent, the emotional deprivation of both parents because of the illness, or the intense responsibilities of helping to care for her siblings. Sherry's cup was "dumped," not from abuse but from unintentional neglect. As an adult, her Centers of Balance were not full and therefore she was ill-equipped to deal with life in the most effective manner.

When Sherry left home to live on her own, something she had looked forward to, she was shocked as her life began spinning out of control. Sherry attended college and began putting on weight. She attributed the weight gain to "the freshman 15" and didn't worry too much about it. By the time she graduated, however, she was 40 pounds heavier than when she started college. She accepted a job as an Admissions Director for a local university. Although very efficient at work, she found herself isolated when she wasn't working. She was confused and lonely. As her weight continued to creep up, she became more and more unhappy. She had a series of unfulfilling semi-romantic relationships, but felt so badly about herself that she would not allow herself to get close to anyone she dated. People at work noticed a marked difference in her demeanor.

She was grumpy much of the time and began to isolate herself at work. Before long, she realized she was turning into a bitter, lonely woman, and she was only 29 years old.

Sherry admitted that food had become her only source of comfort over the years. Eating was the only activity she looked forward to. She longed for the end of the workday so she could go home to a nice quiet evening with ice cream and brownies. Weekends were spent between the couch and the refrigerator. She was miserable, and she knew it. She attributed all of her misery to the fact that she had become obese. When she was 120 pounds over her healthy weight, Sherry had bariatric surgery at the urging of her physician. She initially followed all of her surgeon's instructions. She lost 115 pounds in the 16 months following surgery. She regained 10 pounds, but was comfortable with that.

At 26 months post-surgery, however, Sherry had gained another 30 pounds, which is when she sought therapy. She reported that she found herself eating the same foods that gave her comfort before surgery. She had settled into many of the same negative behavior patterns that she had engaged in before the surgery.

As I worked with Sherry, she caught on quickly. I helped her to recognize that she had entered the adult world with a half-full cup – and not because anyone had treated her badly. Emotional and physical neglect, being burdened as a child with the responsibility of her younger siblings, and the loss of her mother, had dumped a significant portion of Sherry's emotional wellness, leaving Sherry fairly empty on the inside.

Once on her own, loneliness engulfed her. Sherry had been used to having her siblings around. They had provided her with company and, more importantly, with a sense of purpose. They needed her. On her own, there was no one who needed her, except when she was at work. Lonely, grieving, and without a sense of personal purpose, Sherry used food to try to fill herself. Like some people use alcohol, other drugs, gambling, or excessive shopping, Sherry used food to try to fill internal voids.

Sherry quickly understood that she was using food to try to stabilize the imbalances within herself. She was able to recognize that no amount of food could satiate the grief she felt over her mother's death. Instead, she came to understand that she could talk about her loss and cry about it with friends or in therapy. She understood that she needed to find healthy purposes to fill the void left from no longer feeling needed by her siblings. Sherry got busy with a variety of volunteer activities and continued in therapy to work on her grief issues. She was able to see that unless she worked toward rebalancing her Centers of Balance, she would remain less than full and likely to turn to food for solace.

Intentional Neglect

Neglect can be unintentional, but it can also be deliberate. When a parent chooses to leave the kids at home alone so she can go to the clubs, neglect is a deliberate choice. When parents are too caught up in their own careers, social lives, or partners to tend to their children's needs, neglect is a deliberate choice. Putting their own needs above the needs of their children is an indicator of the imbalance and emptiness on the part of the parents. The absence of adult attention and supervision in the lives of these children sucks the "good stuff" from their cups. Does this mean these parents are "bad" people or "bad" parents? Not necessarily. It does mean they are making parenting decisions that will adversely affect their children.

Abuse

Research has shown that childhood sexual abuse is frequently a factor in obesity. Sexual, physical, and emotional abuse powerfully disrupt a child's Centers of Balance. Abused people are often very close to empty by the time they reach adulthood. They try to cover their hurt, shame, pain, and rage in a multitude of ways, often turning from one negative behavior to another. Food is frequently a favorite choice for abused people. They don't have to share it. They can be with this treasured friend, food, all alone where no one can bother them. Food doesn't hurt them in the moment and if they're lucky, there is an abundance of it. The emotional pain endures, but as long as there is food, there is temporary solace.

"I knew that my overeating was related to having been sexually abused," said Shanna. "I just didn't know how to stop feeding my face. Even after my surgery. The first week I was home from the hospital, I ate food I knew I wasn't supposed to because I was so desperate to calm the painful emotions inside me. I finally got into counseling. The more I talked about the abuse and how it has affected my life, the less I felt the pain and the less I punished myself with food."

Shanna had punished herself throughout her adult life in a variety of ways. She struggled to understand why she behaved as she had, often times acting against her own value system. She had been in one unhealthy relationship after another. Men called her derogatory names and would "love her and leave her," but she would go back for more. Then she would swear off men but would find herself sitting in front of slot machines for hours at a time. She said, "Food was the only thing that didn't seem to get me into trouble. I know that doesn't really make sense because I had high blood pressure and the threat of diabetes from eating so much."

Shanna learned that abused children believe they have done wrong. They do not blame the adult who hurt them. The victim develops feelings of intense shame and anger, which they are often too young to comprehend. Rarely do they have the skills to communicate such complex feelings, nor do they have anyone to share them with. The internalized feelings are acted out later in life in self-destructive ways that seem to make no sense.

That is very often the case with people who are obese. A negative experience left them feeling badly about themselves. Food is used to medicate the pain but there is never enough food to make the pain go away. More pain is created from the problems caused by obesity. It is a vicious cycle.

Unlike Shanna, Jacob, 26 and unemployed, had not made a connection between having been molested and his sudden increase in weight when he was in the seventh grade. "Everybody said I was gaining weight because I had hit puberty so I just thought that's what was supposed to happen," he told me. "I guess thinking back, none of my friends gained so much weight at that time. I didn't tell anyone about the sexual stuff that happened with the neighbor. It only took place a couple of times and then he moved away. I started smoking pot around that same time. That didn't help either because I always got the munchies pretty bad which only contributed to my weight gain."

"I had weight loss surgery three years ago because I had gotten up to 335 pounds," Jacob continued. "I kept smoking pot, but still managed to lose 140 pounds. As I started losing weight, I found myself crying sometimes for no reason. I have never been able to keep a job for very long, even though I'm pretty smart. I have always just felt like an all-around loser. I finally went to the doctor and he sent me to a counselor. That led to my going to treatment for marijuana – and alcohol, which I drank to excess several times a week. I learned in treatment that I started using food and alcohol and drugs so young for a reason – to hide from my feelings. That's when I made the connection between the sexual abuse I endured in seventh grade and my abuse of food and alcohol and drugs. I know now that I have to stay clean and sober and use food only as fuel to live. I'm getting ready to go to college now and want to be a counselor after I graduate."

An abuser causes damage to a child and then the child grows up and causes himself damage, often not having any idea why. If an abused child does not make the connection between his or her unhealthy adult behaviors and the painful events that happened in the past, that grown-up child will continue to eat too much or drink too much or smoke too much or shop too much or sleep with too many people or engage in a combination of unhealthy compulsive behaviors. Abuse comes in a variety of forms: physical, mental, emotional and sexual. (By the way, just for the record, spanking is hitting and hitting makes a child feel, well, hit. Being hit makes anyone, adult or child, feel hurt, anger and shame. Hitting a child spills her Cup.)

Criticism: Abuse by Another Name

Overt abuse is hard to ignore. Criticism comes in the direct, overt form: "What's the matter with you? You can't do anything right", "I don't know why I bother with you. You're not worth it", and the old favorite of the hard-core criticizer, "You're a loser."

Name-calling is also overt criticism. "Fatso," "Tub of Lard," and "Hog" are words that obese people know all too well.

But criticism can be equally painful when it's covert, or indirect. At times people aren't sure if they are actually being criticized. For example, if your Aunt Carol says, "There's not a thing wrong with the way you drew that flower, honey. But if it were me, I would have done it this way...", you may not be sure if she was being critical or not. She could be genuinely sweet and kind and trying to show you how to draw better, or she may be indirectly criticizing you, subtly noting she doesn't approve of your drawing.

23

Sandra said her mother, who always wore a smile on her face, could tear through her heart by saying, sweet-as-you-please, "If one wants a thing done right, one must do it herself." Sandra knew she had sorely displeased her mother when she heard those words in that syrupy sweet voice which had the sting of a wasp.

Sandra couldn't understand her own compulsion with food until five years after having bariatric surgery and a weight regain of 80 pounds. She only knew for sure that there was a seething anger inside of her that she could not identify. Food always seemed to lessen her pain. Sandra had worked very hard to lose weight following her bariatric surgery. She was upset about regaining so much back and was devastated by the time she found her way to counseling. In therapy, she completed a thorough family history. She identified that both of her parents were very covert and indirect in their interactions with Sandra and with each other. Sandra was able to produce a substantial list of criticisms she had received as a child and that she continued to repeat to herself as an adult. As she worked through the anger about having been criticized so often during her childhood, she began to take her excess weight off. Sandra learned not to use food to try to conceal her emotions.

Abuse by Comparison

Often, comparisons can erode a person's self-esteem. Comparisons, too, can be direct or indirect. "Why couldn't you be more like your brother?" is the direct form. "I wonder how it might work if you tried to do the project the way Billy did?" is a subtle, but also stinging form. A constant diet of comparison leads to inner turmoil, a lack of self-confidence, and anger toward the person to whom you are being compared. These feelings, if left unacknowledged or unexpressed, are directly related to overeating and other unhealthy behaviors in an attempt to "not feel." For a surgical weight loss patient, the consequences of repressing negative feelings are regaining weight, continued unpleasant feelings, and possibly switching to another unhealthy behavior.

Abuse by Chaos

Brain imaging scans have now proven that the brain development of children who grow up in chaotic environments are different from the brain scans of children who are raised in calm environments. It is not surprising that children raised in calm environments have, overall, healthier and more efficient brains than children raised in homes where there is fighting or other forms of regular chaos.

Brandi's home was "a verbal battleground." She often hid in her room to avoid fights between her parents or her older siblings and her parents. Bags of chips, cans of soda, string cheese, and chocolate bars were Brandi's constant companions. She could avoid the fear and anger she felt toward her family by literally stuffing herself. Food remained the greatest source of stress-relief in her adult life. Ironically, she chose working in the stock market industry, an unbelievably chaotic environment.

Brandi monitored the ups and downs of stock trading on her computer with the chips, sodas, cheese, and chocolate at her side. Her career choice may have been a subconscious way to recreate the chaotic life she was so familiar with and to perpetuate her negative eating habits. Unless Brandi is able to acknowledge and express her feelings related to living in a chaotic home, she will continue to turn to her trusted calorie-filled friends to ease her emotional pain.

Less Than Full is Less Than Full

Regardless of how a person ends up with cups that are not full and misaligned Centers of Balance, it is imperative to find healthy ways to rebalance. When we feel incomplete, we turn to unhealthy means to fill the void. For bariatric patients, their primary means of doing so before weight loss surgery was food. After surgery, unless they seek to discover what voids their overeating was attempting to fill, they will either turn again to food and regain their weight, or they will find an alternative negative substance or behavior. For 30 percent of those people, that alternative is alcohol.

Abuse by Another's Addiction

Edward's dad was an alcoholic. He never physically abused anyone in the family. However, as the saying goes, "Alcoholics don't get married and have families – they take hostages." Edward and his sister were victims of their father's drunken rantings about what a mistake he made in marrying their mother and how horribly his life had turned out. The kids lived in constant fear of their father's moods, his monologues, and his insistence that he could drive after drinking. Edward grew up fearful of his father, angry about the way his father spoke negatively about the family, afraid because his father would often drink and drive, and sad because he never had a close relationship with his father. Edward was fortunate to know prior to having bariatric surgery that he needed to deal with his thoughts and feelings about his father so he would not return to unhealthy eating behaviors after the surgery. He did not want to continue to use food to quiet the noise of emotional pain, which calls loudly for attention.

Having a parent who is active in an addiction, whether to alcohol, drugs, shopping, gambling, sex, or food, creates a wellspring of negative emotions for a child, even when that child is an adult. Weight loss patients who are children of active addicts are at high risk for regaining weight or acting out in other negative ways until they deal with their own feelings about their parent's addiction.

The Blame-Shame Game

Obesity is a symptom of underlying issues, a sort of nonverbal SOS. But who's to blame for the cause of the distress call?

"You can blame my parents," Haley said. "They called me 'Dumpling' all my life, not because it was cute but because I was soft and chunky. They embarrassed me in front of relatives and ordered for me in restaurants, telling the waitress that if I ordered for myself I would have pancakes with ice cream for every meal. It is their fault I'm so fat," she insisted.

Haley was 36 years old, owned her own home, worked as a computer programmer, and did volunteer work, writing grants for non-profit organizations. She left her parents home at age 17 to attend college and has never lived under their roof again. She was a very intelligent, capable woman.

Eventually, Haley softened to the truth that at the age of 36 she was completely responsible for the condition of her body at the present time. In therapy, she identified the issues her parents were responsible for which had a negative effect on her, including name-calling, humiliation, and making choices for her that she was capable of making for herself. She shared her thoughts and feelings with her parents, holding them accountable for their behavior. Yet she could not blame them for the fact that after living on her own for 19 years, she was obese. She had to take personal responsibility for her own choices and her own behaviors. She had to accept personal accountability. The issue is not one of fault, but of accountability, responsibility and dealing with "what is."

In your case, as someone who is actively trying to keep excess weight off, "what is" is that you have made a decision to change your life for the better. You have taken responsibility for knowing you need to save your life.

I Had a Perfect Childhood

The evaluation process before bariatric surgery involves the completion of a personality inventory. Nearly half of my clients complete the inventory in a "defensive" manner, attempting "favorable impression management." Obese people are unaware of, or guarded against, allowing themselves to acknowledge the problems in their lives and their buried emotional pain. This makes perfect sense. That's what they have used food to do: guard themselves from emotional pain.

Rochelle insisted that neither her parents nor her childhood experiences had anything to do with her being obese. An intelligent, accomplished woman with a 10-month-old son and a husband of three years, Rochelle said the reasons she was obese were that she was "too lazy" to exercise and she "loved to eat." It took time for Rochelle to work through her defenses before she was able to acknowledge that her role in the family had been to be "the perfect child." She slowly disclosed how angry she had been with her parents who insisted she participate in "the right" clubs, organizations, and activities. Rochelle had wanted to be a professional ice skater, but her parents said there was "no future in that," in spite of Rochelle showing early talent in skating. Instead, her parents enrolled her in gymnastics and Girl Scouts, and later "made" her be on the debate team and join the church choir. Rochelle attended pharmacy school at their insistence as well. Her parents were always able to convince Rochelle that "they knew what was best" for her. Voicing her opinion during her youth led to lengthy periods of being "grounded," so she kept her thoughts to herself. After beginning her adult career, Rochelle gained weight at a rapid pace. She eventually reconciled her sadness and anger about not getting to follow her own dreams. Her weight finally stabilized.

Sick and Tired of Being Sick and Tired

When you made the decision to have bariatric surgery, you were, as they say in Alcoholics Anonymous, "sick and tired of being sick and tired." You were sick of the way you felt. Tired of the fatigue that came from carrying excessive weight. Tired of the negative ways you were treated by others and sick of feeling the way you felt about yourself. You alone know the depth of the physical and emotional hell you experienced as an obese person. The decision to have bariatric surgery was a decision that you made over time, following failed attempts at weight loss in the past. Diet after diet, weight loss drug after weight loss drug. Hopes up. Hopes dashed. Weight down. Weight rebound. Finally, enough became enough.

After having weight loss surgery and *finally* staring Happily Ever After right in the face, you hear it. That pesky, irritating, bothersome voice you so hoped the surgeon would find and remove during your surgery. You do your best to do what you have done millions of times in the past. You try to ignore it. But it persists. "What if the surgery doesn't work?" You get busy. "I've never been able to keep weight off before. No matter what I did." You get busier. "I know I said I would do 'ANYTHING' to lose this weight but I really hate exercise and I REALLY, REALLY, REALLY miss my chocolate." Fear sets in. "How am I going to survive the family reunion next month with the ribs and the chicken and all of the cakes and pies and brownies and Aunt Rita's cheesecake?" You panic and look for somewhere to turn. Instinctively, you turn where you've always turned when you want to ignore the unpleasant: you turn to the refrigerator. Now what?

Now – use this book! Like a wise grandma, this guidebook will help you gain insight by gently pushing you to look deeper into yourself than you may feel you have the courage to do. You will be comforted and bolstered; you may even be scolded or given a lecture or two. Most importantly, however, you will be *celebrated* as you reclaim your authentic self – the self Grandma saw when you were first born into this world – before the burden of obesity hid your light from shining. Grandma knows that God sent you into this world with a full cup. It got spilled along the way, resulting in a rift between you and your spiritual truth. Obesity negatively impacted your Spiritual Center and now all of life is off kilter.

Help is on the way. Beginning on the very next page, in fact. And this time, no one can stop you! *Eat It Up! Eat It Up! Eat It Up!*

EAT IT UP!

Chapter 3

God Help Me - Really: Your Spiritual Center

"The hunger can be quieted inside and out only when one knows God on the inside."

-- *Author unknown*

Imagine a daisy. Brilliant, individual yellow petals each affixed to a central, strong core. Exquisitely designed and perfectly content in its completeness. Likewise, our Centers of Balance are constructed with five petals attached to a nucleus, the core from which the petals bloom. Our Spiritual Center is that core, the focus, the midpoint, the origin from which the other Centers blossom and to which they are affixed. Consider what would happen if a field of daisies was stricken with a malignancy that eradicated the center of each individual flower. Every single petal from every single flower would fall to the ground or blow around aimlessly in the wind.

The center of a healthy flower holds the petals firmly attached, giving them a place from which to show off their individual beauty. On the ground or blowing in the wind, the petals are undefined. An individual petal represents a part of something larger, but it is impossible to formulate an accurate representation of the whole flower from a single petal.

Like a daisy without the core, a person without a healthy Spiritual Center is incomplete. The daisy without a strong, healthy center cannot nourish its petals. A person without a healthy spiritual center cannot fully nourish the cognitive, emotional, physical, social and enterprising "petals."

Devoid of a healthy Spiritual Center, we become desperate, attempting to find the fulfillment that leads to a peaceful, harmonious existence within ourselves and with others through external sources. Our ability to be our authentic selves is clouded by self-focus and other-focus. The search is exhausting and futile. The only way to find joy and contentment and to live as the person we were intended to be is through a connection with our Creator. Obesity drastically interferes with the ability to remain in tune with God. Obesity inhibits our ability to nurture our relationship with God.

If you are obese or have ever been obese, I ask you to remain patient and open-minded as you read further. You are likely to become angry with me. I am perfectly okay with you being mad at me, realizing it will be one of many times this will happen as you read further. I had a very wise professor one time who repeatedly told the class, "Do not hear what I am *not* saying." I will remind you of this throughout the book. In the pages that follow, I am NOT saying:

- (I am NOT saying) that you have no connection at all with God
- (I am NOT saying) that every obese person fits into a neat little category and has every negative trait, attitude or behavior discussed throughout the book; some of what is written will pertain to you and some of it will not.
- (I am NOT saying) that you are a completely selfish person who thinks of no one else (in fact, you may do just the opposite and think only of others... what you will find out, however, is that the practice of focusing only on others is as unhealthy as complete self-focus).
- (I am NOT saying) that you are a "bad" person in any way, shape or form (I say this because obesity often accompanies low self esteem and having low self esteem frequently means people feel criticized or like they are being told they are "bad" if they receive anything less than positive feedback).

Let's talk about that daisy again. The petals of a daisy receive their sustenance through the core. If the core is diseased, the petals cannot be fed. If our relationship with God is damaged, our ability to nurture the relationship with ourselves and with others is negatively affected. Obesity results in our core, our connection with God, being damaged and impaired. How? Obesity and low self-esteem go hand in hand. Low self-esteem and a positive relationship with God rarely co-exist.

Most people who believe in God believe that we were created in His (or Her or Its) Image. Most people conceptualize the image of God as representing unconditional love, goodness, joy and beauty. If you believe that you were created in the image of God and therefore represent unconditional love, goodness, joy and beauty, there is no room for low self-esteem. Research clearly shows that obese people have low self-esteem. Low self-esteem is not compatible with an intensely close relationship with God. Low self-esteem does not allow you to believe that you are unconditionally loveable, or that you have tremendous goodness, joy and beauty. Typically, when I am alone in my office with an obese patient, they tearfully acknowledge feeling "less than" other people. Less loveable, less happy and less beautiful. Does this mean they hate everything about themselves? Of course not! It does mean that consciously or subconsciously, they have distanced themselves, to some degree, from God.

Cynthia, a 32-year-old married mother of three, told me, "I grew up in a very religious family. I love God and feel He has provided many blessings in my life. It was hard for me to think that being obese had distanced me from God. At first, I rejected that idea completely. But when I got really honest with myself, I realized it was true. I constantly put myself down with negative self-talk. I was jealous of the other moms at my kids' school who were slim. I talked badly about them to try to make myself feel better. Sometimes I was mean to the other ladies without intending to be. I felt sad and angry when they talked about going for power walks together or about shopping for new clothes. I hated exercising, and going shopping was a miserable experience for me. I found myself making sarcastic comments to them about the evils of exercise and shopping. This behavior never helped me feel any better about myself and sure didn't help to build relationships with them.

"One day," Cynthia continued, "it occurred to me that treating others badly was not a way to deepen my relationship with God. I was ashamed of my behavior and figured God wouldn't be too pleased by it, either. I also realized that when I talk badly about myself, it must be upsetting to God. He made me in His image, which is beautiful. For me to criticize and berate His creation must be hurtful. I would never berate my kindergarten son's works of art – his creations. I finally got the connection between my obesity and how it distances me from God – and also from myself and from other people."

Obesity separates us from God and from the person we were divinely intended to be. Matt did not become obese until he was in his late 20s. "I had always been a bit overweight," he said, "but after I stopped playing softball and my girlfriend broke up with me, I guess I got depressed and really let myself go. I slowly gained weight over a period of three or four years until I was nearing 300 pounds. The more weight I gained, the less I interacted with other people. I blamed them for excluding me from events because I was fat. The truth is, it was me backing away from others. I felt miserable. I started hating myself. I stopped being 'the friendly person who always included others' that God created me to be. I no longer accepted myself and assumed others were no longer accepting me. I got mad at God, actually. I accused Him of abandoning me during a hard time in my life. God never abandoned me. I abandoned God. I abandoned myself, and I abandoned others. Food took their place."

When obese adults get mad at God because they are obese, they are failing to take responsibility for themselves. "I was so mad when my therapist talked to me about 'taking responsibility' for my obesity," said Amanda, who has lost 113 pounds since having bariatric surgery. "I was mad at God for a lot of things, and being obese was one of them. It wasn't my fault my parents fed me poorly; I was born to parents who neglected their health and the health of their children! It was easy for me to talk about how irresponsible my parents were, and God did nothing to intervene. I was so angry! It took a lot of work with my therapist before I was willing to acknowledge, that now, in my adult life, I am making similarly irresponsible choices about what I put into my mouth and how much I choose to exercise. I need to be responsible for asking God to guide me in making healthy choices and giving me strength to follow through when I get discouraged or lazy or when I feel hopeless. Today I ask God for guidance and strength every day. I no longer blame anyone else for the choices I make."

God, self, and then others. That is the order of importance most of us learned in our childhood. And it makes good sense in our adult lives. God has to come first. Our relationship with God is where our strength originates. People often get angry with, or blame God for abandoning them when the chips are down. An old Amy Grant song asks, "How do I know there's a God up in the Heavens? Where did He go in the middle of my pain?" It is understandable to wonder where God is when lives are lost in earthquakes and other natural disasters. It is difficult for us to fathom that God would allow the butchering of human life by other "humans" that takes place on this planet every single day. And how do we make sense of God "allowing" a child to be beaten or an innocent person to be raped? We will probably struggle with these questions throughout our lives. We were each given the gift of free will and like all gifts, the gift of free will is sometimes abused. The poem Footprints In The Sand, written by Mary Stevenson in 1936, provides perhaps the best answer to the question, "Where did you go, God, when I needed you?" The last line of the poem is, "The Lord replied, 'The times when you have seen only one set of footprints in the sand, is when I carried you.'" God carries us when the burdens in our life are too much for us. He helps us deal with devastation and loss. Think about when God has helped you through something that you did not think you could bear. It's likely you can think of several instances.

Trying to live without the strength provided by your Higher Power is like trying to build a high-rise building without bricks, glass, concrete, or metal. It can't be done. We need God. We need a daily, ongoing relationship with God. This means talking to God throughout the day: "Dear God, HELP ME! I crave something with a ton of sugar and know that if I eat it I will be SICK! Please help me remember that I have a list of 50 things I can do to distract myself when these cravings hit. Give me the strength to follow through with one of them. With your help I can do this." Just talking to God will slow you down and give you time to remember that you have healthier choices than eating that ton of sugar.

But you may need to make peace with God before you feel comfortable re-building your spiritual relationship. This could take the form of an internal dialogue, or writing a letter to God and then burning it so its message travels through the universe, or talking to a church leader such as a priest or minister or rabbi. Mark recalled making peace with his God the night before having weight loss surgery: "I distinctly recall sitting in my living room the night before I went to the hospital. I had been so angry with God because I was fat. I knew I must take full responsibility for my choices and my health," he said. "I had tried to lose weight over and over and over and every time I gained it back. To successfully lose the amount of weight I needed to lose, I knew that I was going to need spiritual help; help to make healthy food choices and to incorporate exercise into my routine. Sitting my living room, I made the commitment to take responsibility for myself and to turn to God regularly for strength and guidance. I prayed for help to let go of the negative thoughts I struggled with so I could remain positive about myself and about the process of living healthy. I asked for help to accept the love, support and guidance I so badly needed."

Without God, the petals of the flower that make up your life will simply scatter in the wind. With a Spiritual Center holding everything together, you can nourish all aspects of your being.

Balancing Self-focus

This book is all about balancing your Centers, beginning with your Spiritual Center. Once you truly make God the center of your life through ongoing communication with Him, you need to work on balancing your relationship with yourself.

Getting carried away with focusing on the self is an easy and common thing for obese people to do. Obese people are extremely self-focused. Be honest with yourself… When you are obese, you worry about what other people think of you, you wonder what they say about you, and you are hypervigilant about people looking at you. You refrain from going to certain places in public in order to avoid feeling scrutinized. Every day people tell me they hate how kids look at them or point at them or blatantly talk aloud about how fat they are. I hear stories from my obese patients about their angry thoughts and feelings as people stare at them in restaurants and in airports. They shed tears relating the tales of clothes shopping and the dread of having to do so. These are all examples of self-focus, which, in and of itself is not necessarily a bad thing. Everyone is self-focused. What matters is the outcome of that behavior. For obese people, the outcome is often negative and detrimental.

Mary, who lost 135 pounds three years ago following bariatric surgery (which she has kept off), said, "When I was heavy and went out in public, I thought everyone was looking at me thinking negative things about me. I could just hear them calling me ugly names. This led to a horrible negative spiral of thoughts, feelings, and behaviors for me. I would begin reprimanding myself, telling myself that no fat pig like me should go out looking like such a slob. Then I would remind myself how much I hated myself."

After surgery, Mary said, she is still self-conscious but has more balance. "I no longer obsess about people looking at me when I'm in public. If I think someone is looking at me, I remind myself that no matter what they think about me, it is how I feel about myself that matters. Then I talk to myself about what a great job I have done in the past three years in all areas of my life. I remember that regardless of what others think about me, God loves me, I love myself, and I have several people in my life who truly love me, as well. This results in my feeling good about me which translates to my being happier and nicer. Bringing God to the center of my life has helped me work toward balancing all areas of my life."

Of course, it's human for us to think about ourselves. We all do it. The secret is balance: loving and caring for yourself in healthy ways and refraining from being overly self-focused in unhealthy ways. It's likely you have developed a habit of being overly self-focused as an obese person, but you may be unable to recognize the habit. Ask yourself the following questions:

1) Am I avoiding a person or situation because I am worried about what someone else will think about how I look/act/ etc.?

2) Am I neglecting responsibilities to my family, my job, my budget, etc?

3) Is my behavior attracting negative attention?

If you answered "yes" to any of these questions, chances are you are focusing too much on yourself. Taking time to exercise and caring that you look presentable in public is a healthy self-focus. Missing your child's school play because you assume others will negatively judge your appearance is negative self-focus. Enjoying being the center of attention at a party for a few minutes can be fun, exciting, entertaining, and good for your ego; part of healthy self-focus. Creating a scene or being raucous at a party because you *need* to be the center of attention at all times is obnoxious and shines like a neon sign that says, "I feel badly about myself."

Consider how you can re-balance your focus. For example, rather than missing your daughter's violin solo because you don't want to be seen in public, remind yourself that her need for you to be at the concert is more important than your shame about the way you look. Instead of going out with the girls for the third time in a week, remind yourself that while your need to socialize with your friends is important, so is your family's need for time together.

Negative preoccupation with self can persist following bariatric surgery. "Even after my surgery, I woke up and immediately thought about what the number on the scale would be. I spent most of the day focused on what I would eat and when I would eat it," Lisa shared at a bariatric support group meeting. "At home I spent a lot of time on the treadmill and lifting hand weights. The amount of time I spent sorting through my clothes was ridiculous, and I'm ashamed of how much time I spent on the computer talking to others who had weight loss surgery. Finally, my kids and my husband had an intervention of sorts with me, telling me they were angry with me for neglecting them. They were excited for me but sad, too, because I didn't act like I cared about them any more. I'm so glad they had the courage to talk to me about how they were feeling."

As you lose weight after surgery, it's normal to get caught up in the excitement of the changes taking place. There are a lot of things to think about. You need to be sure you follow your nutrition guidelines, get enough protein, take vitamins, chew and chew and chew and remember not to drink with meals! You chart what you eat and when you exercise. You plan your meals. You shop carefully for groceries. You have to shop for new clothes because those old "fat clothes" start to fall off. The weight loss and accompanying activity is like a full time job! No wonder you become self-focused! Ask God to center you, to grant you discernment and balance, and to have a healthy self-focus.

Involving your loved ones is one way to maintain some balance during this unbalanced time in your life. Teach them about the Centers of Balance. Demonstrate for them the importance of having God at the center of your life so you can nurture the other areas of your world. Have your kids plan menus and grocery shop with you. Let them help pick out new clothes with you. Let them take turns being your "scribe" to maintain those food and exercise journals. Be creative! Have some fun! This weight loss business can become too serious with all of the "shoulds, oughts, and musts" you are instructed to do!

God, Self, and Finally, Others

It's an irony that in spite of the tendency to focus too much on self, an obese person really loses touch with himself, his true self. The genuine inner person with many God-given gifts is lost in preoccupation with weight-related issues. This affects how the obese person deals with others. As the writer Eckhart Tolle has said, "When you lose touch with yourself, you lose yourself in the world."

Charlie let people take advantage of him all the time, going along with almost anything other people wanted for fear of losing them as friends. His Spiritual Center became grossly imbalanced as he participated in activities contrary to his personal values in an effort to "fit in." Marlene overextended herself on committees at work so people wouldn't talk badly about her. Trina ended up with stress fractures in her shins because she feared if she sat down to rest at work, her co-workers would complain about her. Philippe volunteered to be the designated driver five nights a week so he would have "friends" to go out with.

Charlie, Marlene, Trina and Philippe lost themselves by trying too hard to be part of the crowd. They lost touch with their God and their inner selves in a desperate attempt to be accepted by peers. Other obese people go to the extreme of avoiding contact with outsiders as much as possible. Randy almost lost his job because there were so many days he called in sick so he wouldn't have to face his co-workers. Maria quit a high-paying sales position after she gained a significant amount of weight and took a desk job so she wouldn't have to interact with people. Mika kept her job and took her children to all of their activities, but she stopped participating in any social activities of her own and refused to join her husband in social activities of interest to him.

Without continually making God the center of their lives, obese people, whether before or after surgery, remain off balance. They lose the connection with their source of insight and power, the source to give them the strength to stay on track and follow through, in balanced fashion, with the focus and activities needed for success in keeping their weight off and success in their life.

Balance comes from looking inside yourself to see what your needs and wants are and then finding healthy ways to get those needs met, starting with your Spiritual Center. Bariatric surgery will not automatically restore balance to any Center. Like losing weight and keeping it off, establishing balance in your Spiritual Center and every other Center requires effort! You *must,* however, work toward balance in your Spiritual Center in order to achieve balance in the other Centers. The Spiritual Center is the core of the Daisy that is your life. Feed it and watch the petals that are your other Centers of Balance bloom and grow! Continue to engage in your food addiction and you will see your world, and your connection to God, self, and others fade away.

Food/Eating: an Addiction?

"Minds are like parachutes - they only function when open," noted Professor Thomas Dewar. The word addiction often scares or angers people, but don't slam the door to your mind shut yet. Read each category that follows, and give yourself a point for each statement you answer "Yes" to.

Category One: I often eat large amounts of food or eat for long periods of time or frequently throughout the day.
- I have additional servings even if I'm no longer hungry.
- I often eat more than I intend to.
- I take larger servings than I plan to.
- I eat even though I am not hungry.
- I eat even though I finished a meal recently.
- I eat at meals *and* frequently between meals.
- I am a grazer.

Category Two: I have a persistent desire to lose weight or have made several unsuccessful attempts to lose weight.
- I have started many diets.
- I have lost weight on diets but have regained the weight.
- I regularly say (out loud or to myself) that I want to lose weight.
- I have referred to myself as a "yo-yo dieter."

Category Three: I spend (or have spent) a great deal of time or effort in activities necessary to obtain food, to eat food, or to recover from its effects.

- I have gone out in the middle of the night to get some food I simply had to have.
- I have purchased more than one meal at a restaurant or drive-thru (maybe even asking for a second drink so the cashier thinks I am buying food for additional people), even though all of the food is for me.
- I have done things like drive around looking for the "HOT" sign at the donut shop, indicating there were fresh, warm donuts available.
- I have snuck food so others don't know I am eating it.

Category Four: I have given up important social, occupational, or recreational activities because of food.

- I have made special dates (with myself) just to eat as much of my favorite food(s) as I wanted.
- I have stayed up at night after everyone has gone to bed just so I could be alone to eat.
- I have missed work or other responsibilities so I could be by myself to eat as much as I wanted to.
- I have missed work or other responsibilities because I was sick from eating too much.

Category Five: I have continued to eat rather than doing the work it takes to lose weight despite knowing I have a persistent physical problem that is likely to have been caused by, or exacerbated by my weight.
I have one or more physical problems caused by, or made worse, by my weight, such as:

- High blood pressure.
- High cholesterol.
- Diabetes.
- Knee or joint pain.
- Sleep apnea.

Category Six: I need an increased amount of food to feel full or to achieve whatever the desired effect of food is, OR in spite of eating the same amount of food as usual, it no longer satisfies me in the same way it used to.

- Sometimes I keep eating even though I am full because I am trying to feel better in some way.

Category Seven: I feel like I go through withdrawal if I am not able to eat when I want to, whether I am hungry or not, OR I use another substance besides food (cigarettes, alcohol) or engage in another behavior (shopping, gambling) to deal with my feelings or circumstances.

Add It Up

If you said yes to the main question (or to any of the examples in each category) for **at least three of the categories**, then you meet the criteria for Substance Dependence as described in the Diagnostic and Statistical Manual (IV), published by the American Psychiatric Association. They define addiction as "a maladaptive pattern of substance use leading to clinically significant impairment or distress, as manifested by three (or more)" of the criteria described in the categories above.

People don't like to be referred to as an "addict." The word has such a negative connotation. People tend to think of an addict as a gutter drunk, a homeless heroine junkie, or a "crackhead" prostitute. The reality is that addicts come in the form of janitors, cardiologists, psychologists, garbage collectors, stay-at-home moms, English teachers, judges, accountants, nurses, cashiers, and every other profession. All races, the old and the young, male and female; anyone can be an addict.

An addict is a person whose use of a chemical (including alcohol or food) or whose behavior (eating, gambling, shopping) causes recurrent problems in a variety of areas of their life – in their health, in their relationships, at work, at school, or in other areas of responsibility – and yet they continue to use the chemical or engage in the behavior. (Some would say that addiction is present when a substance or behavior has "gotten out of control" but this definition seems too general to me.) When I say "problems," I mean serious and ongoing issues. For example, this person is an addict: she gets a DUI – a month after sitting on the boss's lap at the company party - just two weeks after having a huge fight with her spouse about how her behavior changes around men after she drinks too much.

I'm also talking about problems such as having spent too much money on a new wardrobe after you have maxed out three credit cards, and after you told your spouse you had already cut up the credit cards. I'm talking about overeating on Thanksgiving and continuing to overeat daily while gaining more and more weight after your doctor tells you that you are on the verge of developing Type II Diabetes, after he told you two months ago that you had developed high blood pressure, which happened after he already told you that your cholesterol was dangerously high. Problems that continue after you are already aware that the substance or behavior has caused problems…those kinds of problems indicate addiction.

Approximately 30 out of every 100 people who have bariatric surgery "switch addictions." Some post-surgical people start drinking and continue drinking even when serious problems arise as a result. Some start spending money irresponsibly even after financial problems arise. Some start having sex with almost anyone. And many others regain their weight because they return to their "drug of choice" – food.

Whack-A-Mole Additcion

One of my favorite games at the fair has always been Whack-A-Mole. If you have never played it, you really should. In fact, maybe all people who are recovering from any sort of addiction should invest in a home-version game of Whack-A-Mole. It would be a great thing to do instead of eating AND it would also serve as a great way to release anger in a healthy way. Just whack away at those infuriating little moles as they pop out of their holes. I digress…

The Whack-A-Mole game has a table-top-like surface with several holes in it. The player holds a mallet in her hand, ready to strike. The goal is to whack the head of a little mole that pops up randomly in one or another of the holes in the table top. The more moles you whack in a certain amount of time, the better you do. This game is the perfect analogy for switching addictions.

Let's say, conveniently, that you are a food addict. Your addiction to food is represented by one of the moles in the game… the "food addiction mole" now has its head above the table. Let's now say that you decide to have bariatric surgery, which means that you are going to whack that little mole's head and he disappears underneath the table top. If all you do to lose weight is have bariatric surgery and do not engage in any of the other healthy behaviors needed for sustained weight loss (exercise, food diaries, portion control, etc.) it won't be long before another little mole pops his head out of another hole on the Whack-A-Mole table top. This mole may represent drinking: it's the "drinking mole." You are no longer eating in a destructive manner, but have substituted alcohol. You are now drinking to numb yourself from painful emotions the way you used to eat to numb emotions. Let's say that your family members mention that you are drinking too much. They are uncomfortable with that and are worried about you. You don't want to be an alcoholic, so you pick up the Whack-A-Mole mallet and whack that "drinking mole" back down underneath the table top. When yet another mole pops up, you are curious. What now? Well, if you still haven't figured out that you are using "other things" like you use food, "other moles" will continue to pop up. This time it's the "spending mole." In no time you realize that you have maxed out your credit card. You look at that mole head above the table top and tell him in no uncertain terms that you are in control and that he is not going to win this round. Two more maxed credit cards later, out comes the mallet and away you go, whacking at that little "spending mole." Before you even put the mallet down, up pops a "gambling mole." This cycle will go on and on and on unless you have the courage to recognize that you are literally replacing one addiction with another. Whack-A-Mole Addiction!

Change is hard. Old thought patterns, feelings, behaviors, and habits are worn into your brain like tire tracks in wet mud. But you can change your negative thoughts about yourself to positive thoughts about yourself. It can be done. *It can be done*. You can also change your negative, destructive behaviors into positive, life affirming behaviors. It takes a lot of work and a lot of re-balancing. ***It can be done.*** Re-balancing your Spiritual Center is the place to start the re-balancing process.

My Pet Peeve

I have a dog that I named Peeve. The dictionary says that a peeve is a source of annoyance or irritation. I named the poor little thing Peeve before I knew his behavior would certainly be a source of annoyance – at least to my husband. Steve did not want another animal in our house, but he felt sorry for me because my beloved dog, Cy, was hit and killed by a garbage truck. My daughter came up with the name Peeve because even the idea of another animal irritated my husband. My furry little friend does, indeed, annoy Steve, but Peeve is loving and special to me.

The bariatric patients I work with are also very special to me. In the pre-surgical bariatric evaluations, when I ask, "What are you willing to do to lose this extra weight and to live a healthy life?" almost every patient tells me, "ANYTHING." I always hope they are willing to follow through with as much vehemence as they have when they declare that intention. At the end of the evaluation, I give each patient a sheet of paper that lists ten specific behaviors that, IF THEY DO THEM, will result in their being successful.

For the post-surgical bariatric patient, success means keeping weight off over time, maintaining healthy eating choices, engaging in regular physical exercise, and living a healthy lifestyle. My list, which I call the GDEs (Gotta Do Ems) of Sustained Weight Loss Success (discussed in more detail in Chapter 8), includes:

- make consistently healthy food choices (protein first)
- maintain portion control
- exercise on a daily basis
- drink plenty of water throughout the day, but not with meals
- eat breakfast
- plan your meals and follow your plan
- keep food and exercise journals
- get plenty of sleep
- utilize a healthy support system (support group meetings and on-line support)
- participate in individual and/or group counseling for at least a year

My annoyance and irritation (my pet peeve) with post-surgical bariatric patients arises because the above list, which holds the keys to a sustained healthy weight and healthy lifestyle, is rarely followed. I know how hard it is to stick to such a list. When I went through treatment myself for my alcohol and codeine addiction, I was told by the professionals and people who had been through treatment before me to do a few, specific things - and I did them. No questions asked. These were the tried and true successful behaviors done by countless others who had sustained sobriety for years and years. If these were the proven tools, then I was going to use them. I followed the advice of people who had been down the road before me and were living successful, clean and sober lives.

Your doctors, the nutritionist, the people who have had weight loss surgery and have kept their weight off, and now me – we are all telling you the secrets of success! It is up to you to carry them out. No one can do the work for you; on the other hand, you can't do it alone. Use the support of others who have had weight loss surgery and follow the directives of the professionals involved in your process! CHOOSE SUCCESS! Turning to God and asking for help and guidance makes the process easier.

Letting Go and Letting God

The phrase "Let Go and Let God" is familiar to those in alcohol and drug recovery circles. As Mary Kupferle, author of *God Never Fails*, wrote:

"Accept the reality that God's wisdom is ever present and available, ready to fill you with new understanding, light and life. Let God fill every void, every emptiness that seems to separate you from the desires of your heart. Let go! Let God fill your need. …Whatever your life experience appears to be, you have, at this moment, an opportunity to let go of personal striving and let God move in you and through you to fill every need.

Tell yourself again and again: I let go. God will fill my need.

Let go. Let God fill your need. Let the creative process of God begin now to fill every point in your life that needs the touch of His great love and healing power. God is ready to do what you cannot do by yourself."

Addiction Shuts the Door on God

When you are active in an addiction, be it food, alcohol, other drugs, sex, or shopping, God is not your priority. In addiction, the substance or behavior you are involved with – (yes, as in, "have a relationship with") – takes priority over God, self, and others. I imagine you're bristling as you read these words. I can hear your arguments. "My kids come before anything." "I would never put anything before God." "My relationships with my family members come first in my life."

We'll talk about denial and other defense mechanisms in the next chapter. For now, think about how your relationship with food interferes with all of your relationships. Earlier you may have acknowledged how you stay up alone at night to eat rather than going to bed to snuggle with your spouse. When you are obese, you don't have the energy or physical capability to participate in many physical activities with your family members (yet, you continue to engage in the behaviors that reinforce your obesity; you somehow muster up the energy to go out in the middle of the night to find a "HOT" donut sign). You have said demeaning and negative words to and about yourself in relation to your obesity. Your health is compromised in many ways.

All of these things are insults to the Creator who wants us to treat our bodies and minds as the miraculous gifts they are. Eleanor Powell noted, "What we are is God's gift to us. What we become is our gift to God."

Back to Where We Started

Your obesity has caused imbalance in your Spiritual Center. Regaining that balance will be a process that occurs over time. You will need to put forth consistent effort talking to God, asking for His help and the help of your family and friends. It takes practice to "let go and let God." You have to learn to put your faith in God, trusting that He will give you strength to make the changes necessary to do the Gotta Do Ems so that you can take your weight off, keep it off, and work toward balance in all your Centers! Once you begin to find balance in your Spiritual Center, you can start focusing on your thinking, on keeping an optimistic attitude and on maintaining positive thoughts, the subjects of the next chapter.

Chapter 3: End of Chapter Exercises

Balance Brainwork
A Personal Review of Your Spiritual Center
Relationship with God and Spirituality

What has obesity cost you in terms of your relationship with God or your spirituality? Write a paragraph describing what God and/or spirituality has meant to you in the past. Has God/spirituality played a major or minor role in your life? What role would you like for God/spirituality to play in your life in the present and in the future?

Relationship with Self

Make a list of 10 words you typically use when you think about yourself (*not words you use to describe yourself to others*, **but words you say – either inwardly or out loud - about yourself**.) Are these words positive, neutral, or negative? What purpose do these words serve in your life?

How have you hurt yourself by being obese? What are three ways you plan to improve your relationship with God and three ways you plan to improve your relationship with yourself as you lose weight and keep it off? List four ways you have been negatively self-focused as an obese person. Identify four specific ways to eliminate negative self-focus.

Relationship with Others

Write a paragraph describing the five most important people in your life and the reasons they are important. How have you hurt or neglected these important people because of your obesity? List five ways you plan to improve your relationships with these people as you improve your health and lifestyle.

Balance Busters

Read each of the following thoughts out loud, paying attention to what you are aware of in your body – how you feel. For example, do you feel a knot in the pit of your stomach? Does your chest feel heavy? Do you feel muscles tighten? Are you sad? Scared? Angry? Then read the reframed statement and do the same – pay attention to how your body feels.

God hasn't helped me out during all of the bad times I have had.
OR
Sometimes it's hard to feel God's presence. I will make the choice right now to ask for His guidance, trusting He will provide it in the way He sees fit.

God doesn't answer my prayers.
OR
I will be patient, knowing God sees the bigger picture and believing He answers my prayers in the way that is ultimately best for me, even if I can't see it in the moment.

I feel too guilty and ashamed to ask God for help because I stopped turning to Him for help a long time ago.
OR
I can turn to God at any time knowing His love for me is much greater than I can understand. I will ask Him now to give me strength to make healthy choices today.

Write examples of negative thoughts you have related to God, to yourself, and to others that interfere with making healthy choices in your life. Then write a reframed statement that is more positive that will lead to making healthier choices. Throughout your day, when you become aware that you are making negative statements, make the active, conscious choice to reframe and restate your thought to something more positive. You will feel better and choose positive behaviors.

Balance Boosters
Write a list of three positive behaviors you will incorporate into your daily life to keep God at the center. For example: I will begin each day by reading a page from my favorite devotional book.

List four ways you will honor your Spiritual Center each day. For example: At the end of each day, I will remind myself of a God-given talent I have used in a positive way such as, "Today I used my gift of empathy to console my co-worker whose son is having marital problems."

List two ways you will ask others to help you keep your Spiritual Center balanced. For example: "I will ask my sister and best friend to gently inform me if they see me overextend myself/not set healthy boundaries by saying 'yes' to everything others request of me."

The Best of the Best

The ideas and thoughts below are gleaned from writers and thinkers who can add to your repertoire of positive thoughts and behaviors:

- "Every evening I turn my worries over to God. He's going to be up all night anyway." - Mary C. Crowley
- "Diseases of the soul are more dangerous and more numerous than those of the body." – Cicero
- "Health is a state of complete harmony of the body, mind and spirit. When one is free from physical disabilities and mental distractions, the gates of the soul open." - B.K.S. Iyengar
- "People see God every day, they just don't recognize him." - Pearl Bailey
- "When we can't piece together the puzzle of our own lives, remember the best view of a puzzle is from above. Let Him help put you together." - Amethyst Snow-Rivers
- "God enters by a private door into each individual." - Ralph Waldo Emerson
- "God's promises are like the stars; the darker the night the brighter they shine." - David Nicholas
- "Say you are well, or all is well with you, And God shall hear your words and make them true." - Ella Wheeler Wilcox

Cardinal Convictions

Write three Cardinal Convictions, or positive thoughts, that you will incorporate into your daily life to balance your Spiritual Center on a continual basis. For example: I have God with me at all times as a source of constant support and strength.

Chapter 4

I Think I Feel: Your Cognitive and Emotional Centers

"You must start with a positive attitude or you will surely end without one."

-- Carrie Latet

Healthy eating and healthy living behaviors following bariatric surgery depend on the balance of your Cognitive and Emotional Centers. These centers share the focus in this chapter because cognitions (thoughts) and feelings (emotions) are inextricably linked, and are closely followed by behavior. What you think affects how you feel. What you think and how you feel affect how you behave.

Let's play a game. Think about, or jot down, your first thoughts and reactions to the following topics:

- Abortion
- The Superbowl
- Slavery
- Feminists
- The Homecoming Queen
- Harley Riders
- Physical Exercise

The thoughts and emotional reactions about these topics are as varied as the number of people reading this book. There are no "right" or "wrong" responses. Your particular thoughts and feelings about each topic are the results of your experiences with them and what you were taught by others. For example, a person raised in a strong Catholic family is likely to think negatively about abortion and possibly feel sad and angry about it. These responses may be the result of five previous generations of devout Catholics passing on those messages, or these ideas and feelings may develop after studying the Catholic religion in one's own adult life.

Avid football fans likely look forward all year to Superbowl Sunday. Their Superbowl enthusiasm may be the result of a lifelong tradition of celebrating that day. It may be the result of having played football themselves, or they may have developed a passion for it later in life, perhaps because of a loved one who plays or loves the game.

Many people view "Harley riders" as a group of rough-looking, solidly built men with long hair. They may fear these "hoodlums" and avoid them at all costs. Others admire the men and women from all walks of life who are passionate Harley riders.

Clearly, the thoughts we have about any topic influence our feelings and in turn, our behaviors. Consider this domino effect:

Thought: "I think exercise is a waste of my valuable time."

Feeling: "I feel angry that my doctor and family members constantly lecture me about how I need to exercise."

Behavior: "I refuse to make time for something I hate."

Consider this alternative thought, feeling, behavior pattern:

Thought: "Exercise is really important to my overall health and well-being. Exercise is essential in order for me to keep my weight off following bariatric surgery."

Feeling: "I'm scared about exercising because it is new to me; yet, I'm excited about getting into it because of the benefits."

Behavior: "I exercise even when I don't feel like it because it is important for me in so many ways, especially since having bariatric surgery."

The thought-feeling-behavior pattern depends on you. *You choose your thoughts!*

Choosing Your Thoughts

James didn't understand the concept of choosing his thoughts. "My thoughts just are!" he declared. "I'll be driving to work and all of a sudden I'm thinking about something random. Thoughts just pop into my head... I might start wondering if my in-laws will stay with us for the Fourth of July. I didn't *choose* to think about that while I was driving to work."

James is right. Thoughts may "just pop into" our head, but when this happens, *we then choose* what we do with those thoughts. For example, James could choose to elaborate on his thoughts as follows: "Wow. I hope my in-laws don't stay with us when they come to town. They have three other kids who live here. Why don't they stay with them sometimes?" Jim feels frustration related to his in-laws and their visiting habits. If he chooses to continue this line of thinking, his irritation will increase, and he is likely to act out those feelings when he gets to the office. His behavior will reflect his internal anger and the first person to greet him with a "good morning" may get an angry grunt in response.

James could, alternately, decide that thinking about his in-laws' potential visit is a waste of time: "I'm not going to think about something that may or may not happen – especially when July is four months away! Besides, I just get upset thinking about my wife's parents. I'd rather remember how sweet the kids were when I left home this morning." By making a conscious choice to end a negative train of thought and replace it with a more positive one, James feels better and acts more kindly toward others.

As he prepared for bariatric surgery, I asked James in a therapy session to talk about the thought-feeling-behavior interplay he experienced in relation to one of his recurrent thoughts about food: "Food is the only thing I can count on to be there for me, no matter what."

When I asked James how he felt when he experienced that thought, he replied, "I feel angry because neither of my parents was there for me when I was a kid. I came home alone from school and stayed by myself almost until bedtime. I used food to help me feel less lonely. In my adult life, my wife isn't there for me. Sure, she's home, but she stays in one room watching TV, and I stay in another. I keep my chips and salsa right there with me, and I'm not so lonesome."

"When you feel angry and alone, what do you do?" I pressed.

"I eat. I sit in the room by myself feeling mad and lonely and think about how I wish my wife would ask me to join her or wish she would come and join me."

Here is the domino effect of James's thoughts, feelings, and behavior:

Thought: "I couldn't count on my parents to be there for me. I can't count on my wife to be there for me. *I can count on food to be there for me.*"

Feelings: Anger and loneliness because people did not provide him with comfort.

Behavior: Continued isolation and overeating leading to more anger, sadness and loneliness.

James did not like it when I suggested that he *chooses* to think about food as a friend and uses his sadness and anger as *excuses for not accepting responsibility to make positive changes*. As a child he needed the presence, love, guidance, support, and nurturing of his parents. As a child, he was powerless to change the fact that they left him alone for so many hours at a time. As an adult, however, being angry with his wife and thinking of her as abandoning him was an excuse to cling to food and not take responsibility for getting his needs met. As an adult James could *choose* to ask his wife to join him or he could *choose* to join her. If she is not interested in either option, he could join a bowling league or other social activity to find companionship.

You *can* choose to alter your mind in positive ways, but you first need to learn to recognize what you currently do with your thoughts. If your thoughts are negative, you can dwell on them (if you want to feel badly.) You can opt to find a more positive way to frame the thoughts (thereby feeling better). Your behavior will follow suit, depending on whether you focus on negative or positive thoughts. As William James said, "The greatest discovery of my generation is that human beings can alter their lives by altering their attitudes of mind."

Balancing the Cognitive and Emotional Centers

Balancing your Cognitive and Emotional Centers is a learned behavior. If you are an obese person, you have probably not learned to *consciously choose how to think* so that you feel and behave in healthy ways. Most of us consider our thoughts as being unconscious. A mentor or therapist can help you learn the skills of paying attention to your thoughts and consciously choosing to focus on the positive aspects. These are essential skills for sustaining weight loss following bariatric surgery.

Thought "Habits": Learned Behavior?

We have thoughts and feelings about people and things based upon what we were taught and based on our experiences. "My mother had me on a diet since I was eight years old. She took me to Weight Watchers when I was ten. I lived my entire life thinking about what diet I was currently on or which one I was going to try next. I hated the word 'DIET' and still feel angry just hearing it spoken aloud." "My dad was the most pessimistic man on the planet. He found something wrong with everything: haircuts, sunny days, rainy days, winning the lottery, you name it. Now my wife says I sound just like him." "Grandma always said I would end up fat just like her. Now I am fat and tell everybody I ended up just like Grandma said I would." These are examples of comments I hear from patients every day. *Children are taught thinking habits.* Watch and listen to preschoolers "play" and you know exactly how their parents think and act.

I worked at Head Start for a time and watched 4-year-olds play with dolls. Some would cuddle their babies, smiling and cooing at them. Others scolded them and repeated words I knew came straight from mom or dad. When my husband and I taught a class for teens at our church, it was the same thing. Kids would profess staunch opinions on very adult topics. Again, I could hear the parents' voices coming from the mouths of these teens.

What thoughts did you learn from your parents? What are you teaching your children about how to think?

Learning to be Judgmental

You are judgmental! That's right. Judgmental. I'm not calling you names... everyone is judgmental. The word may sound negative, but each of us makes judgments each and every day. Your thoughts and feelings about a person or a topic are your judgments about those things. We make "judgments" in order to make decisions. For example, I personally judge skydiving to be a terrifying thing to do and have no plans to engage in that particular behavior. Saying that skydiving is dangerous and terrifying is a judgment, but it is not "judgmental" in the common use of the word.

"Being judgmental" has negative connotations. To "be judgmental" suggests that a person makes a seemingly authoritative, definitive decision about a person, a group, or a thing. We often go around talking like we have be-all and end-all knowledge. "Those cheerleading, Homecoming Queen types are all the same: ditzy, rich, snotty stuck up little girls who have everything handed to them on a silver platter." "You know how those red-necks are with their pickup trucks and their can of snuff and their huntin' gear." "Everybody knows that all surgeons are egomaniacs." "All those good-for-nothing welfare people just need to get off their rears and go get a job." "Depressed people just need to pick themselves up by the bootstraps." Be honest. How many of these judgmental stereotypical statements have come from your own lips? If not these, I am certain you have spoken in a negative, authoritative manner about some group or topic, be it gays or lesbians, a minority culture, a religious group, or a political candidate.

The obese people I work with regularly talk about the frustration they feel when others judge them as being "lazy, irresponsible, stupid, ugly" or any other number of derogatory terms. Ironically, these same obese people can behave in some extremely negative judgmental behavior themselves. In the groups I conduct with post-surgical bariatric patients, I often point out the judgmental comments participants make. Often the comments are geared toward other groups of people with difficulties (ironically somewhat like their own).

"I just don't understand why someone would ever make themselves throw up after eating." "If someone wants to stop drinking, why don't they just stay away from the bar? Why don't they just refrain from buying alcohol? Why don't they just drink lemonade?" "I would never put something as dangerous as cocaine into my body." The people making these comments are not intending to sound mean or cruel or harsh. They usually aren't aware that they are being critical and judgmental. When someone points out that their comments are judgmental, they quickly realize how they engage in the very same negative behavior they despise when it is directed toward them. Most of their judgmental comments are based on thoughts and ideas they had grown up with. Their judgments come from not understanding the particular problem they criticized.

So it is with those who judge the obese. Non-obese people don't understand how anyone "could do that to themselves," or "let themselves go like that." Non-obese people haven't been in the shoes of the obese and truly cannot understand the thinking, the emotions and the behavior surrounding obesity.

The important points are:

- Everyone (including you, the reader) judges unfairly.
- No one likes being on the receiving end of negative judgments (including you, the reader).
- Most people easily identify when others are being judgmental but are unaware of their own judgmental comments and behavior (including you, the reader).

STOP IT! Start right now focusing on your own thoughts, feelings and behavior. Let others worry about theirs. Put effort into trying to see life as though you were in another's shoes. Admit that you can't fathom being in that person's shoes and therefore have no right to judge them or their situation.

Wouldn't it be nice, as an obese person, for someone not familiar with being obese to get inside your head for a day to know the torment you go through? To have them understand how food consumes your thoughts and how you hate it and often hate yourself? To hear the horrific things you say to yourself about how you look and feel? To really feel the pain associated with being stared at and mocked? Maybe then people wouldn't be so cruel.

Can you, as an obese (or formerly obese) person imagine what it's like to be an out-of-control drunk and truly hate yourself for knowing you are letting your family down day after day after day but you can't seem to get the car to drive straight home after work because it keeps taking you to the local watering hole?

Do you, as an obese (or formerly obese) person, genuinely know the despair associated with not being able to get out of bed in the morning or to be unable to swallow a bite of food because your depression is that incomprehensibly deep?

Are you capable of understanding an uneducated, minority girl's lack of self-esteem which prevents her from knowing how to fill out an application or believing she is capable of holding down any sort of job after she has been called "worthless and stupid" all of her life and having been told she will "go nowhere?"

Probably not.

Stop focusing on how unfair the judgments of others are toward you. Choose not to judge and to ignore the judgments of others. Think positively and you will feel better. Your actions will follow suit. You will treat others more fairly and will be treated more fairly in return. As one of my favorite motivational speakers, Zig Ziglar says, "When you choose to be pleasant and positive in the way you treat others, you have also chosen, in most cases, how you are going to be treated by others."

It Gets Worse

Now that we have established the fact that we can all be "judgmental" in the most negative sense of the word, allow me to point out something equally dismal. As miserable as it is that other people negatively judge obese people, and that obese people negatively judge others, the fact is: The obese person judges herself even more critically than anyone else possibly could.

Think about the things you have said to yourself lately. I'm betting there have been comments like, "You idiot!" "Why did I eat all of that?" "God, I'm so stupid. How could I have done that?" "I'm such a loser" "What was I thinking?" "I'm ugly." "I'm fat." Most of us don't run around sharing those thoughts out loud, but we often have an ongoing narrative of negative comments about ourselves streaming through our brains. Our negative self-talk can be like a train that has no caboose - it never seems to end.

Here's a challenge I pose to clients and am now presenting to you. I ask you, "Would you say the negative statements above to your very best friend?" Think about it. Your lifelong soul-sister calls you up, four months after having bariatric surgery and says to you, "I can't believe what I did today. A co-worker brought in my favorite chocolate fudge cake and throughout the day I managed to eat three pieces of it. I feel horrible... physically and emotionally." Is this what you would say to her: "Wow! You're really a loser! How stupid can you be? I can't believe you let yourself eat three pieces of chocolate cake after what you have been through! What were you thinking?"

Come on now. You would never in a million years do that to your best friend! More likely you would say something along the lines of, "I can hear how upset you are with yourself. I know you are feeling horrible right now. Let's talk about it. You have been really diligent about what you have been eating since you had surgery. Your health is important to you. Eating that cake obviously wasn't in your best interest. It's not like you have regularly overindulged like that since having your surgery. There must be something going on. What was bothering you?" You would *kindly* talk to your friend about the circumstances surrounding her eating too much cake. You would help her remain accountable for her behavior, but you would not beat her up for it.

The challenge to you is to treat yourself as kindly as you would your best friend. This includes talking to yourself as gently as you would your best friend, even when you need to hold yourself accountable. In other words, when friends come to us, they are looking for affirmation and validation of their feelings. Good friends want to be supported and encouraged by the people they love and trust. They also want to be gently held accountable for their behavior. The second response above is one that demonstrates good listening and good friendship skills. You can practice these same skills of good listening and good friendship with yourself as well as with those you love.

Frances, a 29-year-old hairdresser worked very hard to improve her self-talk, especially when she "screwed up." "My mom was a single parent who worked a whole lot when I was a kid," said Frances. "She didn't have much patience for us kids when she was at home. She grew up in a loud Italian home where folks didn't pay much attention to how nicely they talked to each other. So when any of us screwed up, Ma would say things like, 'What'd ya do that for, you good-for-nothin' kid?', or 'Can't you do anything right?' I heard that so often I really didn't think I *could* do much right. And the kids at school called me 'tubby' and 'dummy.' I didn't realize that I, too, talked badly about myself until I was in group therapy with other ladies who also had bariatric surgery. They started pointing out that I called myself 'idiot' and 'numbskull.' So every time I would say something bad about myself in group, I had to find a way to say it more positively. Now I talk nicer to myself and about myself, and I feel better about myself."

Try this: say to yourself, "I hate the way I look and feel. I hate the way people stare at me." Pause. Pay attention to how you feel when you say those sentences. Sad, mad, scared, angry? Say it again: "I hate the way I look and feel. I hate the way people stare at me." Pause. How do you feel? Where do you feel it? You may notice a tightening in your chest or in your abdomen. Did you find your teeth clenching as you read the words? Was there a lump in your throat? Did those words evoke frustration? Irritation? Sorrow?

Now say this: "My physical appearance is improving since I have been taking better care of my health. It's nice to hear the kind things people say as they notice." Again, pause. How do you feel? Optimistic? Hopeful? Grateful? Pleased? Where do you feel it? A lightness in your chest? A tingling in your stomach? A smile on your face?

I'll say it one more time: *What you think affects how you feel.*

The following statements are comments I hear frequently from bariatric patients. Read them to yourself or out loud. As you do, pay close attention to how you feel emotionally and to the sensations in your body. Say:

- "I try to stay at home most of the time because I'm embarrassed to be seen in public." (Pause, pay attention to how you feel and where you feel it.)
- "It's not fun to eat in a restaurant, especially when I'm with other people. I think other people are watching to see what I eat." (Pause, pay attention to how you feel and where you feel it.)
- "People think I'm a happy person. I tell others I'm a happy person but I cry a lot of the time when I'm by myself. I don't really like myself." (Pause, pay attention to how you feel and where you feel it.)
- "I've lost and gained weight so many times in the past. I always end up gaining it all back, plus more. I'll always be 'the yo-yo dieter.'" (Pause, pay attention to how you feel and where you feel it.)
- Now, read the altered, more positive, versions of these sentences below. Again, pay attention to how you feel emotionally and to how your body responds.
- "I have stayed at home most of the time because I've been embarrassed to be seen in public. I am going out more now because it reminds me that I am as worthy as everyone else in the world. Getting out is also good incentive for me to continue my healthy habits. I like going places and feeling

better about myself." (Pause, pay attention to how you feel and where you feel it.)

- "When I eat in a restaurant, I worry that other people are watching to see what I eat. Instead of hating that others are watching, I have decided it's a good thing because it reminds me to make healthy choices. Who knows? Maybe I'll inspire others to eat better, too!" (Pause, pay attention to how you feel and where you feel it.)
- "People think I'm a happy person. I cry a lot when I'm alone. I haven't liked myself for a long time. Now when I cry I think about the tears as shedding the pain from my inside. When I finish crying, I congratulate myself for letting go of pain and then remind myself of three things that are good about me." (Pause, pay attention to how you feel and where you feel it.)
- "I've lost and gained weight so many times in the past. I always end up gaining it all back, plus more. This time I am choosing to get help, learning how to take the weight off and keep it off, and I am choosing to get support to help me over the long haul." (Pause, pay attention to how you feel and where you feel it.)

Most people feel at least neutral, if not hopeful, when they read the second set of statements. The result of *choosing to think more positively* is not necessarily feelings of complete happiness and joy. You may, however, move toward ending your self-battering and toward a more positive roadmap for your future behavior.

What You Think Affects How You Feel and What You Do

The author Denis Waitley has said, "If you believe you can, you probably can. If you believe you won't, you most assuredly won't. Belief is the ignition switch that gets you off the launching pad." Take the four statements from the preceding section. In each case, the change in attitude and orientation from negative to positive is a catalyst to practice healthier behaviors. You *can* give yourself positive reinforcement in the form of positive thoughts that ultimately results in positive behaviors!

Your Cognitive and Emotional Centers are not balanced when you regularly say negative things about yourself. Picture a child's teeter-totter with 20 negative statements loaded onto one side and no positive statements on the other side. In order to balance the teeter-totter, you must acknowledge positive things about yourself!

Imbalanced Cognitive and Emotional Centers usually tilt toward the negative. New ways of thinking need to be learned *and practiced* to improve your feelings about yourself and to achieve balance.

A Word, or Words, About Feelings

When I went into treatment for my addiction to alcohol and drugs, I was at a loss when the therapists would ask me, "How are you feeling?" One day, after being asked that same damn question one time too often, I lost it. "What do you mean, 'How am I feeling?'" I shouted. "I have no earthly idea what you are talking about when you ask that and you keep asking me and asking me and asking me!" I was obviously (but unknowingly) feeling a combination of anger, frustration, and shame (because I didn't know how to answer the question the "right" way), but I had no words to describe my feelings at that time. I knew how to be angry, but many years earlier I had closed the door to other emotions.

Chances are that as an obese person, you, too, have a limited range of emotions. You can probably fake happy pretty well to the outside world although you are often miserable (either consciously or subconsciously) on the inside. Or maybe you can't even fake happy, but have sadness down to a fine art. You're miserable and everyone around you sees, feels, and hears your misery.

Generally speaking, people who are masters of the angry realm of feelings (irritated, frustrated, grumpy, or downright mean) are avoiding feelings in the sad category (grief, despair, loneliness). Angry people are comfortable with being angry. Sad feelings are terrifying, and yet inside, these people are filled with sadness.

Sad people, on the other hand, are comfortable with being upset, miserable, and tearful but they do whatever necessary to avoid feeling anger. Yet they have the equivalent of a keg of dynamite stored up internally.

Obese people experience the gamut of emotions, although they may think they feel only one or two, or like me, they may not have any idea how they feel. Everyone deals with the four basic emotional categories every day: sad, mad, glad and scared. That's how the counselor at the treatment center categorized feelings for me. He explained that as I became more familiar with feelings, we could add "advanced" feeling words like "concerned" (a subset of the scared category), "thrilled" (part of the glad family of feelings), "impatient" (a variety of mad), and "distressed" (a member of the sadness clan). Initially, however, using the four categories of mad, sad, glad and scared was a helpful educational method.

Learning to recognize and name how you feel is imperative in preventing you from regaining the weight you lose following bariatric surgery. *Unless you recognize, acknowledge, and learn to deal with your feelings in healthy ways, you will continue to use food as a means of avoiding feelings and will regain some or all of the weight you lose following surgery.*

As you learn the words that define feelings, start to "listen to your body." You will learn how you physically experience mad, sad, glad, and scared. Remember how you reacted to the statements earlier in this chapter? Some people experience anger with stiff muscles, closed fists, clenched teeth, taut arms, or tightened stomach muscles. Some feel their heart rate increase. Pay attention to your body. Awareness is the name of the change game. By becoming aware of your thoughts and feelings you will be able to make healthier food and behavioral choices. Unacknowledged thoughts and feelings tend to "drive the bus," or, in the case of a food addict, drive the person straight to the refrigerator.

After being in the post-surgical therapy group for seven months and having lost 85 pounds, Melony shared her discovery of how her thoughts and feelings influenced her eating behaviors. "I thought I was emotionally prepared for healthy eating behavior before I had my surgery," she said. "I had gone to several support group meetings and was active with online support. To my horror and amazement, three weeks after my surgery, I put myself through bout after bout of coming home from work and standing at the sink, stuffing food into my mouth until I threw up. My online support friends encouraged me to get into counseling because I was likely to do some real physical harm to myself if I continued that behavior. In group therapy, I didn't say much for the first five or six sessions. Listening to the others, though, I figured out that the 'thoughts and feelings thing' they all talked about was important to healthy eating behavior. I started writing down in a little spiral notebook what I was thinking and how I was feeling on an hourly basis. As I discovered how angry my thoughts and feelings were throughout the work day, I realized that my overeating when I got home was related to the anger. I talked about this experience during group, and they helped me figure out better ways to deal with my anger so I didn't unconsciously eat and eat and eat to try to swallow my emotion. Now, when I am angry, sometimes I holler and scream all by myself in the car instead of eating when I get home. Other days I play really loud rock music and sing at the top of my lungs. Sometimes I call a friend and vent my frustrations while I drive home. By the time I get home, I have addressed my anger in healthy ways and no longer harm myself through gorging, trying to keep the feelings inside."

Michelle, who has attended individual counseling since having bariatric surgery, said this: "It wasn't until I was eight months post-surgery and in therapy that I figured out something really important about my feelings and my eating behavior. The most difficult times for me after surgery were when I was sad. At those times, I wanted the comfort foods from my pre-surgical days: pasta, pudding, and potato soup. In therapy, I learned to recognize my sadness and to ask myself, 'What do I need right now?' The answer was usually – not surprisingly – 'Comfort. I need to be comforted.' I had been using food in an unhealthy attempt to find that comfort. I learned that I can find comfort by snuggling up in a soft blanket and thinking positive thoughts about myself. I can find comfort by calling my best friends who are happy to remind me of the reasons they enjoy my company. It was really hard at first to do all of this work: first, pay attention to my thoughts, then pay attention to my feelings, then try to figure out my emotional need in relation to those thoughts and feelings, and then make a choice about how to meet that need in a healthy way. But it has worked! Sure – sometimes I still think about how nice warm, banana pudding would be when I'm sad. But I remind myself that if I eat to try to cover my feelings with food, I'll still have the sadness and will also be angry with myself for eating. Instead, I tell myself I can find comfort in healthy ways and will be proud of myself for doing so."

The Past Meets the Present

During therapy, Michelle also realized that a great deal of her sadness as a child was related to her mother being out drinking rather than being available when Michelle got home from school. That's when Michelle would turn to the pudding or macaroni and cheese for comfort. She was surprised to discover that she doing the same thing in her adult life in response to sadness.

Not all obese people (or alcoholics or drug addicts or gambling addicts) grow up in dysfunctional homes, but most do. The majority of children who live in dysfunctional homes are well acquainted with fear: fear of being alone, fear of the parents' fighting (verbally and/or physically), fear of a family member being drunk or high, fear of being called names, yelled at, hit, locked outside, locked inside, sexually abused, accused of God-knows-what, blamed for anything and everything, abandoned, and/or neglected. Survival in a fearful environment takes many forms, eating being one of them. The "survival method of choice" almost always acts as a way to smother feelings.

James and Michelle and so many others realize that food was the way they found comfort as children. Food continued to be the means by which they soothed themselves as adults. It can also be the way they opt not to take responsibility for getting their own needs met in healthy ways as adults.

Childhood Survival Tools Gone Awry

Here's an important and difficult truth: The survival tools used in childhood no longer work in the adult world.

Let's look at some other examples. Some children learn to hide and isolate as a means of survival. In a family where kids are picked on or made fun of, it would be smart for a child to remove himself. In a home where there is a lot of physical or verbal fighting, isolating and hiding protect a child from witnessing or experiencing abuse. But when a boy becomes a man and gets married, he often disappears for hours at a time if he senses his wife is angry with him. He often isolates in his at-home office or his workshop for fear of having to engage in meaningful conversation with his wife or kids. This man never learned in his youth to have healthy, connected, meaningful relationships with family members. How would he know how to do so as an adult?

His tendency to isolate or hide, particularly at times of stress, is a default response for him. It served to protect him during his childhood, but it is a disservice to him in his adult life. He cannot learn to have healthy confrontation with his wife if he continues to hide. He cannot learn to engage in healthy behaviors or to have healthy communication with his wife or children if he hides from them. Changing this behavior requires awareness and learning new, healthier behaviors, then choosing to implement them.

Perfection (or the attempt at perfection, since it is an impossible pursuit) is another example of a coping mechanism that serves a survival purpose in childhood but does not work in adult life. Some children attempt to be perfect little people. They may do so for fear of being treated badly like another sibling and to avoid feeling the painful emotions associated with poor treatment. They may attempt perfection to avoid the kind of criticism they see one parent receive from the other. They may do so in an attempt to get much-needed praise and attention. 'Going for the Gold' in every single situation cannot work in adult life. The need to be perfect as an adult leads to exhaustion.

The use of food is the same way. Food may prevent loneliness for a child. Food may be a source of comfort from criticism, a reprieve from a chaotic environment, the single way of maintaining some control, or the one means of indulgence for a child. In adult life, however, the use of food as a coping mechanism will not ultimately meet the person's underlying emotional needs for companionship, understanding, or acceptance. For a child, food may be the best thing they could find at the time. Adults, on the other hand, have the ability to learn what their emotional needs are, to recognize that food will not meet these emotional needs, and to implement healthy coping skills and behaviors to meet their needs. Using food as an emotional pacifier in adult life does not lead to healthy, functional relationships or a healthy, functional life.

It's a sad truth that many adult relationships fail because people rely on childhood methods of survival to deal with their partners. Isolating, being passive-aggressive, turning to food, alcohol, or spending, attempting to be perfect or a people-pleaser, all interfere with healthy adult relationships.

If adults do not deal with past hurts and learn healthy, mature ways of dealing with the feelings and situations called "life," they will remain in a toxic relationship or continue to engage in one unhealthy relationship after another. If obese adults who have used food as their way of dealing with unpleasant emotions do not learn healthy ways to address feelings and to deal with life, they will remain obese or will replace food with another unhealthy behavior or mood-altering substance.

Training yourself to have a positive attitude is a powerful way to deal with "life" in a healthy way. "Attitude is more important than the past, than education, than money, than circumstances, than what people do or say. It is more important than appearance, giftedness, or skill," says pastor and author Charles Swindoll.

The Emotional Volcano

By the time a person reaches the point of needing weight loss surgery, Emotional Centers are very imbalanced. Years of emotions have been buried under layers of fat. When those fat layers start to melt away, people who have had bariatric surgery are shocked at the volcanic eruption of emotions they experience. I try to warn the patients I see for pre-surgical evaluations about the volcanic eruption of emotions they may experience following surgery. Like the naïve engaged couple, they hear me but think that I'm referring 'to those other patients' because surely their recovery will be smooth sailing. I don't say this to be sarcastic. People simply cannot know prior to experiencing something what to expect afterward. And the pre-surgical state of mind believes that all will go smoothly following surgery, both physically and emotionally. In preparing for weight loss surgery, very little attention is paid to the emotional aspects related to obesity or life after surgery. Hence, the need for this book.

One of my very best friends recently had weight loss surgery. She called me the day after the surgery in tears. She was already grieving the fact that she could not eat like she wanted to. The day after she got home from the hospital she was worried about being hungry and what she would do when she experienced hunger. A few days later she was fearful of "being one of those people who went through the surgery and then didn't succeed." I assured her that her thoughts and feelings were normal for having been out of the hospital only a few days.

Weight insulates us against our emotions. As time passes following surgery and the extra pounds dissolve, buried emotions are freed up, maybe for the first time in years. Cindy, now six years post-surgery, currently healthy and happy at a stable size 10, remembered her first year following surgery: "I thought I was going crazy for a while after I had my surgery. When I was heavy I never would have admitted I used food to suppress my feelings. I didn't know it until I was no longer able to eat like I was used to. After the surgery my husband commented on how irritable I had become. My mother and sister commented on how crabby I was, too. I started feeling depressed. I was mostly upset because one of the reasons I wanted to lose weight was so I could be more active with my husband and kids. I found myself not wanting to be with them at all and when I was with them, I was unpleasant. I finally got into counseling. That was the best thing I could have done because I realized how unhappy I had been when I was so fat. I also talked about how afraid I was to not be fat. This led to discussions about the happy and sad things that happened all through my life during various fat stages and skinny stages. Going to counseling was hard. Dealing with my feelings was especially hard. But I learned better ways to deal with all of my feelings than to try to kill them with food. My entire family is happier now. I still go to therapy at times. This keeps me focused on healthy interactions in my relationships and makes eating healthy much easier."

Recognizing and acknowledging feelings, and learning healthy coping skills to address them are vital to sustained weight loss. Harsh as it sounds, if you already knew how to deal with difficult feelings and situations in healthy ways, you would have done so and food would not have been used as a "best friend," which is how so many obese people describe it.

"But I'm not an emotional eater," you are saying. "I don't use food to 'stuff' my feelings. I didn't gain weight until I was an adult, so my weight doesn't have anything to do with past issues." Let's talk about denial and other defense mechanisms.

Defense Mechanisms - Kidnappers of Rational Thought

Defense mechanisms are what we use to protect ourselves from being hurt emotionally. Defense mechanisms can be thoughts or behaviors, and they are most often subconscious. We use these mechanisms to avoid emotional pain. Defense mechanisms include denial, minimizing, projecting, intellectualizing, passive aggressiveness, and rationalizing.

Denial in the Obese Population

Denial is rampant among addicts of all sorts. Addicted drinkers and smokers of marijuana routinely proclaim "I can stop any time I want to." That may be true – for a short time. Many obese people swear they "hardly eat anything." But the indisputable fact is that obesity, except in specific, uncommon circumstances, is the result of an excess of calories in relation to the number of calories burned. Period.

Yet, time after time, the people I interview as part of preparation for bariatric surgery insist that they "really don't eat much." They aren't lying to me. They honestly believe they don't eat much. Realistically, however, they would not be obese if they did not eat too much of the wrong things over a prolonged period of time, without sufficient physical activity to balance the caloric intake. Nor would they lose so much weight after surgery except for the fact that their caloric intake is drastically reduced.

As noted earlier, each potential bariatric surgery candidate I interview completes an extensive personality assessment. The purpose of the assessment is to screen for potential problems that may interfere with their ability to deal with the process of surgery and the lifestyle changes following surgery. For example, if a patient has a severe anxiety disorder, knowledge of this prior to surgery is essential.

In evaluating people prior to bariatric surgery, I rely on the Personality Assessment Inventory (PAI), which was authored by Lesley C. Morey and published in 1991 by Psychological Assessment Resources (PAR). Approximately half the people I evaluate have results indicating that they think of themselves as *"being relatively free of common shortcomings to which most individuals will admit, and are... somewhat reluctant to recognize faults or problems in [themselves]."* In other words, denial.

You may be arguing with me right about now, thinking it may not just be obese people that show half of all PAI responses indicating this form of denial. It is definitely true that persons other than the obese get these results. In my experience, however, in using this instrument with other groups, such as chronic pain patients, that the obese population has a higher percentage of people responding to the instrument in this way. It is also true that surgeons have a "typical" response pattern to personality inventories, as do attorneys, as do construction workers. People in similar circumstances often have similar personality profiles.

While it is certainly true that obese people are not the only ones who demonstrate denial, in my experience, the obese population has a higher percentage of people who respond in this defensive manner. Denial is rampant among the obese as well as those addicted to other substances or behaviors.

Two years after his gastric bypass, Tom reported, "It wasn't until the past six months that I allowed myself to be honest about the kinds and amount of food I ate during the years before surgery. I already felt so miserable and ashamed about how I looked and felt. If I admitted that I ate practically non-stop I would have felt even more hateful toward myself. Now that I have lost 180 pounds, it is still hard for me to admit I ate so much that I made myself sick, mentally and physically - high blood pressure, high cholesterol, diabetes, sleep apnea, you name it. I just wasn't able to say I was doing that to myself because I was unable to stop eating. It hurt too much."

Denial serves another purpose for the obese or otherwise addicted person, as noted by Sharon, who lost 110 pounds following her lap band procedure. "It was hard for me to come to terms with my denial. Staying in denial kept me from having to take responsibility for myself. My therapist had to work with me for months to help me understand that. I get it now. As long as I was able to fool myself into believing that I didn't eat as much as I did, I could deny responsibility for my obesity. I didn't have to admit that I could change my behaviors and accept responsibility for my health. Now I like taking responsibility for what I eat and how much exercise I get. I feel strong and in charge of my life."

Minimizing (Mini Denial)

When a person uses the defense mechanism of minimization, he doesn't completely deny a behavior, but "makes light of it." The purpose, of course, is to lessen the intensity of his emotions. "It was easier for me to say that I 'ate a bit too much now and then' than to admit I gorged myself every day," Samuel shared at the bariatric support group meeting. He encouraged those who had not yet had surgery to get honest with themselves about what they ate, noting that "it makes being honest about other things in your life easier as well. And that makes getting healthier, physically and emotionally, a much quicker process."

Projection: Kinda like Judging

It always made me chuckle on the inside when I worked at the alcohol and drug treatment center and would hear comments like the following, "I know I smoked weed every day for the past ten years, but at least I'm not a crackhead." When I worked at the residential facility for teenage males who had substance abuse issues and legal histories, it amazed me when a young man who was incarcerated for burglary would become infuriated with another resident who stole from him. These are examples of projection.

"In the women's group I attended following my gastric bypass procedure, I used to talk about how little willpower alcoholics had," Michelle shared. "I thought badly of another type of addict and was willing to condemn them for not taking responsibility for themselves, all the while denying my own lack of willingness to take responsibility for my own behavior."

Intellectualizing: Defense of Choice for the Learned

Highly intelligent and/or educated addicts can be especially frustrating at times due to their use of the defense mechanism intellectualization. The word intellectualization just sounds irritating. We all know someone who fits this description. "You can't tell them anything. They already know everything." This is the person who uses intellectualization. Sometimes what they say is completely wrong but they'd never admit it. Furthermore, you would likely doubt yourself when engaged in conversation with them because they sound so good. They sound smart (and usually are). They use words well. They are convincing.

Intellectualization keeps a person "in their head and away from their heart." In other words, they avoid feelings by using words. Sara used this defense strategy to avoid the hurt and anger she felt when she experienced rejection by males. "It is ridiculous that a man cannot love me for who I am, heavy or thin. I have a Master's degree. I have a good job and a nice home. It is simply the fact that society has placed too much emphasis on physical beauty." She would go on long diatribes about the injustices related to her perceived reasons a man was not attracted to her. In group therapy, she initially became indignant when others told her that her appearance is an indication of how she copes with life and

71

how she takes care of herself. After several weeks, her anger lent itself to the sadness and shame she genuinely felt about her appearance. She stopped being so intellectual about the issue. "I just want to be loved. I'm unhappy with how I look and hoped if someone else would accept me no matter how much I weighed I might be able to accept my weight, too."

Rationalization: Excuses, Excuses, Excuses

As a therapist, the excuses I hear from people result in my cycling through feelings of disbelief, bemusement, incredulity, and frustration. (No, I don't forget that I was once a queen of rationalization myself). I use my "firm and fair" philosophy in dealing with people's rationalizations. I feel compassion for them, understanding that they rationalize to keep from feeling badly about themselves. I use a dose of reality to help them recognize that they are making excuses so they don't have to take responsibility for making healthy choices. "I don't have time to exercise" is a favorite rationalization used by obese people, even after they have lost enough weight to exercise comfortably. "You are busy, as most of us are," I acknowledge. "The truth is, however, that we make time for those things that are of most value to us. Your health, you said in your pre-surgical interview, is of the utmost importance to you. In fact, I believe your words were that you would 'do anything' to lose your excess weight and keep it off. Exercise is an essential part of that 'anything.'"

I heard this next example used by a speaker at a Harvard conference. She shared that when obese patients tell her they are not "the exercising type" she informs them that she is not really the "tooth brushing type" but she brushes her teeth anyway. Exercise is a must for those who need to lose weight and want to keep it off. *Not* exercising is *not* an option.

"It's hard" is a rationalization I hear repeatedly. I agree that "it's hard" to do the things you need to do if you want to take weight off and keep it off. I empathize with the fact that learning new behaviors is difficult and giving up favorite foods is difficult. It is especially difficult facing painful emotions related to eating behaviors. The reality is, however, that the majority of obese people have done other, incredibly difficult things. I ask people how easy it was to get through college and their Master's programs. I ask them how easy it is to get their three children up and ready for school each morning and be to work on time themselves. I ask them how easy it has been to live with the shame and embarrassment of being obese for many years. Yes, losing weight and keeping it off is hard. Doing the things it takes to take the weight off and keep it off are choices.

Defense Mechanisms as Survival Tools

The defense mechanisms described in this chapter serve the same purpose as the childhood survival skills described in the previous section. They all help to protect a person from unpleasant emotions. Defense mechanisms, like childhood survival skills, are ineffective in healthy adult relationships. *In order to balance the Cognitive and Emotional Centers, childhood survival tools and defense mechanisms must be recognized for what they are. The feelings associated with the realities of a painful childhood and the feelings related to being obese must be addressed directly. Healthy new coping skills must be learned and specific behaviors must be implemented in order for an obese person to lose weight and to keep it off permanently.*

Defense mechanisms take rational thoughts hostage. They won't release the rational thoughts because, like a kidnapper, if they release the prisoner, they can't get what they want. People use defense mechanisms and childhood survival skills because they want to keep painful emotions at bay. If they give up the denial, the rationalization, the intellectualization, the perfectionism, or the isolation, reality and painful feelings creep up on them. Rather than facing reality and experiencing the feelings, many people continue to exist in the la-la land created by overeating, the use of alcohol or drugs, gambling, or shopping.

A balanced Cognitive Center is dependent on dealing with reality. For the obese person, these realistic thoughts may include:
- "I am an overeater."
- "I do not get enough physical exercise to balance the intake of calories I consume."
- "I eat to avoid feeling lonely."
- "I use food to drown my feelings of anger at my parents for abusing or neglecting me."
- "Food is my way to avoid my feelings of low self esteem."

Balanced, realistic thinking leads to balanced emotions. For example:

73

"I am an overeater. I eat to avoid feeling lonely. I am responsible to find ways to fill the loneliness in my life. Food cannot do that. But I can join singles' groups to deal with loneliness in a healthy way. I can also join a gym, a book club, and participate in numerous other activities. The choice and the responsibility are mine."

Why Do I Do What I Do?

Behavior, as I've said, follows the direction of your emotions and thoughts. One of the tricky things about this complicated, interlaced maze of thoughts, feelings, and behavior, is that a lot of our thoughts are subconscious. And very powerful. That's why our behavior sometimes makes no sense to us. Many bariatric patients want to know "why" they do some of the seemingly senseless things they do. For example, Brianna stood in front of her refrigerator eating everything she could upon returning from the hospital after having her bariatric surgery. She cried as she shared, "I knew I shouldn't be standing at the refrigerator shoveling food into my mouth after I just had surgery. I just didn't seem able to stop myself. Why would I do such a detrimental thing to myself?" Callie, three years post-surgery, continues to binge and purge. "Why do I still do this?" she bemoans.

Why? Why? Why? Before I answer that, let me suggest something worth taking some time to think about. Would having THE answer to why Brianna stood at the refrigerator eating and potentially damaging her body so soon after surgery have given her what she needed to stop that behavior? Would providing Callie THE answer (if there were such a thing as THE answer) help her stop bingeing and purging? Doubtful, on both counts.

Don't get me wrong. I often refer to myself as an "insight junkie." I like knowing the reasons behind what I do. I have learned through my own experience and from working with hundreds of patients, that insight can be helpful, but it is not necessary or sufficient to create lasting behavioral change. Does it help? Probably, in some cases, but let me restate this: Having insight into WHY we do something *may* help us understand ourselves better, but knowing WHY we do something is NOT necessary for us to change our behavior. Nor does knowing WHY we do something necessarily result in a change in behavior.

Let me illustrate through the two real examples above. Brianna worked in individual and group therapy sessions to gain insight and understanding into the reasons she was obese in the first place. She did a fantastic job exploring family of origin issues. She discussed the messages she got from family about her appearance and her weight. She talked about how it upset her that so much focus was placed on how she looked. She shared the family history of eating behaviors. She explored the origins of her self-image, how she came across to others, ways she tried to make up for feeling badly about herself, etc. etc. etc. It seemed there was no stone left unturned in terms of her self-exploration. Brianna did uncover a tremendous amount of information about herself as a child and as an adult.

This knowledge she obtained in therapy helped her understand herself but did nothing specifically to keep her from wanting ice cream or from going to fast food joints. Ultimately, with or without a deep understanding of herself, past and present, she had to make conscious decisions in the moment and accept the consequences of her behavioral choices. In other words, before Brianna attended therapy, she (consciously or unconsciously) often made the decision to drive through fast food restaurants every day and purchase two or three meals to consume by herself. After having surgery and while gaining insight during therapy, Brianna still had to make a decision every day whether or not to go to the fast food restaurant. Insight is not necessary or sufficient to ensure behavior change.

WHY IS THAT?! Why didn't the insight help Brianna change her behavior? Because behavior is often driven by subconscious needs and wants. I know… earlier I said that behavior is the result of a person's thoughts and feelings and now I'm saying that needs and wants determine behavior. They are sort of the same thing. Work with me here. Let's explore Brianna's behavior when she came home from the hospital and stood in front of the refrigerator eating. She said she didn't know why she did that. She knew she shouldn't be standing there eating but didn't think she could stop. This suggests she was acting without much conscious thought. If she had stopped and made her thoughts conscious before she went to the refrigerator and opened the door, her internal dialogue would have gone something like this: "Well, I'm home from the hospital now. There's no one here with me and I'm scared. I'm afraid that even though people said they would help me through this, I will be

75

alone. I'm sad and angry because I hoped my sister and cousin would come over to help me ease into being home. They always let me down. No one really cares that much about me. Why did I have this surgery? Food has always been my friend. I'm going to eat. I don't care."

The reason it's so important to learn to recognize what you feel is so you don't react to those feelings in harmful ways, such as overeating. Not only must you learn to stop and listen to what your thoughts are, you can help yourself learn to make healthy decisions by asking yourself what you need or want (emotionally) in the current circumstance. For example, if Brianna had listened to her internal dialogue, she would have realized that she was scared, sad, hurt and angry. By asking herself, "What do I need or want right now?" she could have recognized that she wanted and needed support and to feel important enough to have her sister and cousin there for her. After realizing what her emotional needs/wants were, she would be able to make a conscious choice about getting those needs met in healthy ways, such as calling someone else to come be with her. Because Brianna did not stop to listen to her thoughts, she was not aware of her needs. She reacted negatively to her subconscious negative thoughts, which led to negative feelings, by engaging in the negative behavior of standing at the refrigerator eating.

Knowing what you need emotionally *can* help you make good behavioral choices. If you take the time to discover what you need, you can choose a healthy way to get the need met before you react in an unhealthy manner. One of the things Brianna came to understand was that she often went to a fast food restaurant to get food when what she really needed was to "feel full" emotionally. Her feeling of emptiness was not about a lack of food. She needed companionship, affirmation, friendship and love. It was these things she needed to fill up on. Being consciously aware of her genuine needs, she could choose to get them met by asking a friend to play tennis, by taking a scrapbooking class, or any number of healthy activities. Even if she did not become aware of her emotional needs, Brianna knows that fast food is not a healthy choice for her. She can choose to make a healthy behavioral choice with or without insight about her emotional needs.

Your thoughts are often subconscious, yet they still influence your feelings and behavior. Your thoughts are the key to understanding what your emotional wants and needs are in a given situation. Therefore, the answer to "WHY DO I DO WHAT I DO?" is… You do what you do in an attempt to get an emotional need or want met.

Don't underestimate the power of long-term bad habits. Brianna had developed years of bad habits. She had been going to her refrigerator and mindlessly eating without conscious awareness of her needs for a long time. For years she had thought negatively about herself. Strive for progress and not perfection while making these changes. But make the changes you must if you want a healthier future. Doing so leads to health, success and happiness. Jim Rohn, motivational speaker and philosopher reminds us: "Happiness is not by chance, but by choice."

A Call for Action

Callie also participated in extensive individual and group counseling after her weight loss surgery. She did a terrific job working through extremely painful childhood issues including sexual abuse. Weight was a constant source of tension between she and her mother throughout Callie's life. Although Callie kept her weight off after surgery, she continued to engage in bulimic behavior, which she had practiced for years before having surgery. She was now a successful business woman, highly respected in her field, yet the painful effects of her childhood still haunted her. Sadly, she acted out her feelings of low self-worth by continuing to binge and purge. The insight she gleaned during therapy, by itself, was not enough to change her behavior. Insight is no match for years of abuse by others followed by years of self-abuse. *Conscious choice, bolstered by positive thinking and a repertoire of new behavioral skills is the only way to triumph over years of negative behavior.*

Acquiring the knowledge of new behavioral skills is only part of the solution. Some people say that knowledge is power, but knowledge by itself does not equal power. Knowledge put into action is truly powerful! Obtain knowledge of new skills, then use your new positive attitude and put the skills into action! The new skills? I'm talking about things such as journaling about your thoughts and feelings instead of going to the refrigerator, calling a friend instead of driving thru the fast food joint, getting on an Internet web site for bariatric patients, knitting, doing the laundry, visiting someone at a nursing home, rocking a sick baby at the hospital, planting a flower, cleaning a closet, doing a crossword puzzle, sending a care package to a friend, writing a long overdue thank you note, practicing the piano, washing a window or floorboard, going to a movie, reading a funny book, contacting a cousin you haven't spoken to in years, calling a friend and volunteering to babysit, going to the gym, staring at the ceiling... anything to divert your attention long enough to prevent you from engaging in unhealthy behavior. Who knows? You may even make someone else's day happier while improving your own.

Remember, insight into WHY you do or do not follow through with healthy behaviors is not what matters. *Doing* or *not doing* the healthy behaviors is what counts. Oh – and "TRYING"... "trying is dying," as they say. You either DO the healthy behaviors or you DO NOT. You either choose to eat a donut or you choose not to. You can't "try" not to eat a donut. You either choose to exercise on the treadmill or you choose not to. You can't "try" to exercise on a treadmill.

Every time you choose a healthy behavior you help balance your cognitive and emotional centers. You think about your options and you choose a positive behavior. This results in your feeling more positive, which in turn, leads to additional positive behaviors. Thoughts, feelings and behaviors...they're connected!

Cognitive and Emotional Centers, Post-surgery

Some of the most common problematic situations for post-bariatric patients include:

- holiday eating
- restaurant eating
- family, office and social eating situations
- grocery shopping
- cooking
- shopping for clothes
- the clothing store dressing room

The list could go on and on. Fortunately, we do not have to address each of these issues individually, as you deal with them all in the same way: Plan your work and work your plan.

First, as you anticipate each of the situations above (and other potentially difficult situations), reflect on: 1) how you thought of each situation in the past, 2) how you felt about each situation in the past, and 3) how you behaved in each situation in the past. For example, Natalie shared her reflections about the holidays, a time of year she was

78

concerned about after having gastric bypass surgery. "I used to love November and December. It meant two months of wonderful eating," Natalie recalled. "I was excited just thinking about mom's pies, Aunt Cecelia's Christmas cookies, and the office holiday party with every fancy hors d'oeuvres I could imagine. I always gained 10 or 20 pounds. I worked hard to ignore the weight gain and refused to spend any time alone during those months so I wouldn't think about how I was harming my health."

Second, consider the realities of how you handled each situation in the past. What were the consequences to you? Natalie said, "I used to eat as a way to keep myself from feeling any emotions for two solid months during the holidays. If I had let myself feel, I would have been ashamed of how I focused so much on the food and less on the holidays themselves and the people I got to see. I would have felt embarrassed and angry about how much I ate. I can clearly see that I chose to remain emotionally numb so I wouldn't have to take responsibility for my behavior. It took a lot of help from the others at the support group to deal directly and honestly with the reality of my thoughts, feelings, and behaviors about holiday eating."

Third, consider each upcoming situation. Choose how you want to think about each situation and how you want to prepare for it. "Since having surgery three years ago, I have learned to think about November and December differently," Natalie continued. "This year, I am choosing to focus on my relationships with family and friends at holiday gatherings. I know there will be a lot of tempting food there. I will give myself permission to *sample* two of my favorites *after* I have eaten a meal of healthy foods in healthy portions. When I am finished eating, I will brush my teeth to have the taste and thought of food out of my mind. I will drink water as I talk with people so my hands are holding something. When I think about the holidays now, I think about them with confidence. I feel excited about seeing my cousins and other out-of-town relatives. I feel optimistic because I have a plan in place to help me deal with this extraordinary eating situation."

Fourth, have support measures planned in advance. Sometimes a person or situation will trigger subconscious thoughts or memories that lead to unexpected intense emotions, followed by reactive behavior, which may involve overeating. It is important to have a plan of action to obtain support in vulnerable situations. "For me," Natalie said, "My plan for support included informing two of the members from my support group that I was attending a family get-together. I obtained their permission to call them if I needed support while at the gathering. I also plan to keep a note card in my purse on which I have written five affirmations to help me stay committed to my plan. Finally, I have given myself permission to leave the event if I feel overwhelmed. These things work for me."

Fifth, process the situation afterward. This may mean writing about it in a journal, talking with a friend, or discussing it in therapy. Be honest about what you were thinking, how you were feeling, and what your behavior was in the situation. If you didn't do as well as you hoped, talk about what happened. Review the plan you had made and discuss where you got off track. Learn from every situation. Find what works best for you and utilize those tools in each potentially difficult situation.

The Balance Thieves ~ Old Tapes

As easy as it sounds to "Plan your work and work your plan," I am aware that yes, it's hard. Each of us must deal with old, negative tapes that play through our heads, for one thing.

Your current age is the amount of time you have been playing a tape inside your head that contains negative messages about you. It may sound like this, "You are fat. You are not loveable. You'll fail at this weight loss attempt. You always do." After living on this earth for 30 or 40 or 50 years, your mind will never be without the messages you have received about yourself throughout your life. You can, however, record a new track onto the tape in your brain. Changing the way you talk to yourself, think about yourself, and feel about yourself requires ongoing effort but doing these things *does* change how you think and feel about yourself, and ultimately, how you act.

Here's how you do it: As soon as you become aware that you are saying something negative to yourself, you think or say out loud, "Stop It!" Or imagine a huge, red STOP sign in your mind. Then change the thought as discussed earlier in the chapter. Say something more positive about yourself. Do this diligently, even when you feel too tired or defeated. Say something positive about yourself. Remember to talk to yourself as kindly as you would talk to your best friend.

Head Hunger

Head hunger can be as real as anything you may have physically felt before. However, "head hunger" is not physical. "Prior to my surgery, I was used to feeling really, really physically full before I stopped eating," Mark said. "If I didn't feel miserably stuffed after eating, I thought I was truly still hungry. Since having surgery, I sometimes long for that really full feeling. To me, this is head hunger." Kristy described head hunger as "the desire I sometimes have to eat, whether I feel physical hunger or not... it's about wanting food. The truth is, my head hunger is about wanting to feel satisfied. Usually I really crave emotional satisfaction, not food." Abigail said, "I had very bad eating habits before surgery. Now, at certain times of the day when I used to eat, I think I am hungry. To me, that's head hunger. It's really just bad habits. I had conditioned myself to associate eating with certain times of day, specific television shows, and when I did things like read."

To defeat head hunger, try one (or more) of the following:

- Talk directly to it: "Okay, here you are again, Head Hunger. Well, what do you want this time? Let me help you figure it out by asking myself some questions. What have I been thinking about? How am I feeling right now? What do I want or need emotionally? What is a healthy way for me to get that need met?"
- Whether or not you are able to identify an emotional want or need, ask yourself: "What is a healthy behavioral choice I can make at this moment rather than choosing to eat?" Then DO that healthy thing!
- Tell yourself that even if you are physically hungry, you have planned to eat at a certain time, and until then, you will choose to drink water so there will be something in your stomach. Remind yourself that you can and will survive feeling hungry.
- Sit down and do nothing for ten minutes. Nothing... including thinking... just breathe. Just BE.

The Committee in Your Head

Taking time to "just be" is something most people have to work hard on! Not thinking can be a difficult task! There will be times when it seems there is a virtual "Committee in Your Head." Not to fret. If you have a "Committee in Your Head" and "hear different voices" does not, in this case, suggest you have become seriously mentally ill. The "Committee in Your Head" sometimes has board meetings as you go about the process of changing from old, unhealthy ways of thinking, feeling and acting to healthier ways of doing all three. You may be walking into the grocery store, prepared list of healthy food items in hand, when all of us sudden a meeting is called to order.

Board Member #1: "Damn! Something in this store smells great. Somebody find out where that delicious aroma is coming from."

Board Member #2: "Settle down. We're not here to go on a scavenger hunt for things that smell good. We are here to purchase the grocery items on our list."

Board Member #3: "I don't know about the rest of you, but I'm getting tired of all of the fruits and veggies. I vote we follow our nose and sniff out the source of that olfactory delight."

Board Member #2: "Stay on Task, #3. We planned our work. Now let's work our plan."

Board Member #1: "Plan, schman. My mouth is watering and we are getting closer. I'm certain I smell fried chicken and biscuits. It has been a long time since my taste buds have danced to those delicacies."

Board Member #2: "You're just gonna have to waltz right on past the deli, Mr. Dancing In the Stars. If you want chicken, there are plenty of skinless, boneless chicken breasts in the meat department."

Board Member #3: "Who said you get to be the boss around here, #2? Seems to me its me and #1 against you and we want fried chicken!"

This is what the "Committee in Your Head" can be like. You argue with yourself. You think about positive choices. You consider unhealthy choices. You waver. You disagree with yourself. Maybe you even argue with yourself. Argue away – just be sure 'the last word' you have with yourself is the one that chooses the healthy behavior or 'the next right thing'. In the grocery store scene, a positive ending would be:

Board Member #2: "All right. Everybody listen up. We had an agreement before we came to the grocery store. We worked hard to prepare a menu and a list before we got here. Let's just do the job we came here to do. If not, the rest of the day will be negatively impacted and we have fun things planned for the day. Come on, now. It's easy to get distracted here in the middle of the store with the food all around and the smells tempting us. But let's get the items on this list and get out of here. We'll be really proud and it will give us confidence that we can get through the next tough situation, too."

Board Member #3: "I know you're right. I got overwhelmed when I saw all the old favorites here that caused us so many problems in the past. I'm on board. Let's get our groceries and go home."

Board Member #1: "That chicken still smells really good. But, okay. Let's go home and grill chicken. That will smell good too and we'll feel a lot better after eating something healthy. Let's do this thing! Good work, gang!"

Triggers and Balance

Grocery shopping can be an emotional trigger that threatens a person's resolve to make healthy choices. Other triggers include going places where they typically eat poorly such as the movie theatre, the mall or the county fair. Eating at restaurants (especially buffets), holiday gatherings, office parties and special social gatherings such as weddings are examples of situations abundant with triggers that could lead to unhealthy eating. Watching cooking shows, reading food magazines, and clipping food coupons are less obvious examples of behaviors that are negative triggers for many people. "I was mad when my therapist suggested I stop watching the food channel. I didn't see how those shows could possibly harm me. What I learned is that when I watch that channel, I really am more focused on food. I think about it. I want to try different recipes. I need to take the focus off food in my life. Not just the food that goes in my mouth, but food in general. If I were an alcoholic, I would stay out of bars because sooner or later I would end up drinking. The same is true for me and food. If I surround myself with recipes, coupons, food magazines, and cooking shows I am making it all the more difficult to get the focus off food in my life. I am experimenting with hobbies that have nothing to do with food and I'm having fun."

Maintaining Cognitive and Emotional balance are important when working toward the goals of sustained weight loss and balance in life. Food triggers act like rain hitting a sand castle to dissolve the foundation upon which our balance lies. Going to a buffet or reading cooking magazines can stir up the Committee in Your Head which awakens old negative thoughts. You know what happens to our feelings if negative thoughts take over. Negative behaviors follow negative thoughts and negative feelings. Therefore, it is essential that you minimize the triggers in your immediate environment and make choices to avoid people and places that have a potentially negative impact on your new healthy life. Cancel your subscription to all food magazines and get rid of all food channels. Stop pouring over cook books and recipes online. Tell your friends you don't go to buffets. Take your own food with you to social gatherings. Do whatever it takes to minimize temptation and to avoid triggers to negative eating behaviors. Bolster and maintain balance in your Cognitive and Emotional Centers.

Thoughts, Feelings, Behavior

"The state of your life is nothing more than a reflection of your state of mind," said Dr. Wayne Dyer. A healthier body will result from your having a healthier mindset. It's true! As you tune out negative thoughts and practice choosing positive thoughts, your attitude will improve. Your more optimistic attitude will lead to healthy behavioral choices which will result in better physical health. Tell yourself, "Exercise is essential for sustained weight loss and better health. I don't always like to exercise but 'It's What I DO' and I love the way I feel afterward. I look forward to that feeling so I get out and walk every day. My cholesterol is at a healthy level and my blood pressure continues to decrease." Think about your physical health. As you do, remember that your thoughts and feelings about food choices and exercise will directly impact your physical health, the focus of the next chapter. Read on!

Chapter 4: End of Chapter Exercises

Balance Brainwork

1) Write a page (or more) about your parents' attitudes/ways of thinking. Was your mother the kind of person who looked on the bright side of things? Or did she tend to be cautious or scared or negative in her thinking? Did your father encourage you to take risks? Did he talk positively or negatively about people and situations?

2) Write a few paragraphs describing how your thought patterns tend to be like your parents' and how your thinking differs from theirs. Are you more or less critical than they were? More optimistic or pessimistic than they were? More or less self-focused than they were? Did they follow through on the things they said they would do? Do you? Did they encourage you and others? Do you encourage or discourage others?

3) Write a "therapeutic letter" (which means you write it but don't send it) to each of your parents and tell them how their thoughts about you and their actions toward you affected how you feel about yourself.

4) Write a page about how your thinking will impact your behavior, especially in your life following weight loss surgery.

5) Next to each of the following descriptions of people, write down your immediate thoughts and feelings related to the person(s)/groups described:
   - a middle-aged man on a Harley Davidson who has long hair and several tattoos on his arms
   - a young woman in clean blue jeans and a white sweater at the grocery store with two young children
   - a young woman with bleached blonde hair wearing a miniskirt and halter top
   - a male in his mid to late 20's wearing ragged blue jeans and a dirty tee-shirt who is hitchhiking on the side of the highway
   - a teen-age male in loose blue jeans and a tee-shirt carrying a skateboard tucked under his arm

- a group of male teens, hands in pockets, walking around the mall together
- a young woman in a business suit, carrying a briefcase, briskly walking through the airport
- a teenage male in a car with huge tires, shiny wheels, and a blasting stereo

Are your thoughts and feelings about these groups positive, neutral, or negative? Are any of your thoughts and feelings about these people/groups potentially accurate? How do other people judge obese people? Are any of these thoughts potentially true about you and/or other obese people?

Balance Busters

Read the examples that follow. Then, for each of the negative thought statements, write down a positive replacement.

For example:

Negative statement: "I don't like protein; I am sick of protein; I'll get my protein later." This negative thinking leads to feelings of anger about "having" to do something you have been told to do. It can also lead to feelings of frustration about being obese in the first place, sadness about the past, etc., which leads to behaviors that reflect the negative thoughts and negative feelings: "I'll eat what I want to, in spite of knowing it is not in my best interest."

Replacement statement: "I may be sick of protein but I love the way I am looking and feeling as I continue to lose weight and get healthier. I am making the choice to continue doing as I was instructed to do because it works and I ultimately feel better when I eat protein first." This leads to feelings of hope and optimism and feelings of accomplishment and self-pride. These positive thoughts and feelings lead to behaviors that reflect positivity: making the choice to eat protein before eating other foods.

Negative statement: "I'm tired of eating the same old things to try to get as much protein as I need."

Positive replacement statement: _____

_____ .

Negative statement: "I hate seeing other people eat the things I want to eat."

Positive replacement statement: _____

_____ .

Negative statement: "Planning my meals takes up too much of my time."

Positive replacement statement: _____

_____ .

Negative statement: "It's not fair that I have to eat differently than the rest of my family."

Positive replacement statement: _____

_____ .

Write three negative thoughts you struggle with on a regular basis and then write positive replacement statements for each.

Balance Boosters

List five ways to remind yourself to keep thoughts positive. For example: "I will tape a note to my bathroom mirror that says 'I choose to make this a good day by keeping my thoughts positive.'"

The Best of the Best

- "Finish each day and be done with it. You have done what you could. Some blunders and absurdities no doubt crept in; forget them as soon as you can. Tomorrow is a new day; begin it well and serenely and with too high a spirit to be cumbered with your old nonsense." - Ralph Waldo Emerson
- "It's not what happens to you that determines how far you will go in life ; it is how you handle what happens to you." - Zig Ziglar
- "Any fact facing us is not as important as our attitude toward it, for that determines our success or failure." - Norman Vincent Peale
- "Ability is what you're capable of doing. Motivation determines what you do. Attitude determines how well you do it." - Lou Holt
- "Attitude is an important part of the foundation upon which we build a productive life. A good attitude produces good results, a fair attitude poor results, a poor attitude poor results. We each shape our own life, and the shape of it is determined largely by our attitude." - M. Russell Ballard
- "Of all the 'attitudes' we can acquire, surely the attitude of gratitude is the most important and by far the most life-changing." - Zig Ziglar
- "Weakness of attitude becomes weakness of character." - Albert Einstein
- "The last of the human freedoms is to choose one's attitude in any given set of circumstances." - Victor E. Frankl
- "The only disability in life is a bad attitude." - Scott Hamilton
- "Nothing can stop the man with the right mental attitude from achieving his goal; nothing on earth can help the man with the wrong mental attitude." - Thomas Jefferson
- "Attitudes are contagious. Are yours worth catching?" - Dennis and Wendy Mannering
- "If you don't think every day is a good day, just try missing one." - Cavett Robert
- "Happiness is an attitude. We either make ourselves miserable, or happy and strong. The amount of work is the same." - Francesca Reigler

- "A person will sometimes devote all his life to the development of one part of his body - the wishbone." - Robert Frost
- "The excursion is the same when you go looking for your sorrow as when you go looking for your joy."
  - Eudora Welty
- "A happy person is not a person in a certain set of circumstances, but rather a person with a certain set of attitudes." - Hugh Downs
- "Become a possibilitarian. No matter how dark things seem to be or actually are, raise your sights and see possibilities - always see them, for they're always there."
  - Norman Vincent Peale
- "There are souls in this world which have the gift of finding joy everywhere and of leaving it behind them when they go." - Frederick Faber
- "Some days there won't be a song in your heart. Sing anyway." - Emory Austin
- "When you come to the end of your rope, tie a knot and hang on." - Franklin D. Roosevelt
- "Perseverance is not a long race; it is many short races one after another." - Walter Elliott
- "If we are facing in the right direction, all we have to do is keep on walking." - Buddhist Saying
- "I may not be there yet, but I'm closer than I was yesterday."
  - Author Unknown
- "Our greatest glory is not in never failing, but in rising up every time we fail." - Ralph Waldo Emerson
- "Don't let the fear of the time it will take to accomplish something stand in the way of your doing it. The time will pass anyway; we might just as well put that passing time to the best possible use." - Earl Nightingale

Cardinal Convictions

Write three Cardinal Convictions you will make part of your daily self-talk to remind yourself that a positive attitude will lead to positive feelings and positive behaviors. For example: "I choose to focus on what I *can* do and then *I do it!*"

EAT IT UP!

Chapter 5

Move It or Don't Lose It: Your Physical Center

United States Dietary Guidelines, 2005: To sustain weight loss in adulthood, a person needs to exercise moderately to vigorously for 60 to 90 minutes daily.

-- Nutrition and Your Health

Consider this list of activities that many people don't "like" to do, but do anyway:

- pay taxes
- brush their teeth twice a day
- write thank you notes
- do laundry
- go to work every day

Think for a minute about other things you do although you don't really "want" to. Some people claim the majority of their days are spent this way. (Recall what you learned in the previous chapter about positive thinking ... perhaps these people need to change how they think about things!)

Think back to when you were contemplating having bariatric surgery. You may have taken a long time to make the decision, thinking surgery was a drastic step. Maybe you made the decision in a hurry, hoping you had finally found "the answer" to weight loss. Most people tell me they struggled with their weight for years so when they finally made up their mind to have a surgical procedure, they were ready to do "ANYTHING, WHATEVER IT TAKES" to lose weight.

During your preparations to have surgery, how many of the professionals along the way mentioned that taking the weight off and keeping it off would require regular, ongoing exercise? (I hope it was all of them.) On our team, the bariatric program coordinator is a nurse with a master's degree. She reminds patients that surgery is a tool and must be used as such by the patient, along with eating the right things and getting exercise. The nutritionist notes the importance of ongoing exercise along with a healthy diet while preparing for surgery, and for a lifetime afterwards. Our surgeons stress the importance of nutritious eating and ongoing exercise at the initial information session, during individual patient sessions, at the support group meetings, and at patient follow-up appointments. The nurses in the hospital stress the need to follow the diet and exercise protocols before the patient returns home. The members of the local support group encourage one another to eat right and to exercise. And you *know* I preach and preach and preach the word about exercising regularly!

Exercise. Say the word out loud. Say it to yourself. How do you *feel* when you say the word? Excited, bored, curious, disinterested, devastated, horrified, thrilled, angry, scared? Brandon, 88 pounds lighter after having gastric bypass surgery, said, "When I thought about having to exercise in order to lose weight and keep it off, all I could think about were the years of hating gym class when I was a kid. I was always the last one picked for teams when we played any sports. I was clumsy and fat, and kids made fun of me. I had to find a different way to think about exercise so I didn't have such a horrible feeling inside when I even thought about it. I started exercising after surgery when I got myself a bicycle and starting riding it around the track at the park. It was level ground so it wasn't hard, which I needed at first. Since I was on a bike, I was able to ride past people quickly, which meant they wouldn't have much time to see this fat guy on a bike. That helped me too. As I started to lose weight, I wanted more of a challenge and so I took my bike out on the streets. My neighborhood isn't exactly hilly, but there were enough small hills to make it a challenge. Before long, I loved riding my bike and I decided to join the local cycling group. That provided me with a way to participate in group activities where I have made some great friends. I have also learned to set realistic goals designed to improve my performance. When I ride my bike, I forget that I am 'exercising' because I'm having too much fun! In the past, I couldn't imagine using the words fun and exercise in the same sentence."

Most of the bariatric patients I interview before surgery are less than eager at the prospect of exercising at all, much less on a daily basis. Let's face it: heavier people feel less like engaging in physical activity. Pain associated with extra weight decreases enthusiasm for, and willingness to engage in, exercise. Low levels of physical activity increase negative thoughts and feelings about self. The result is a perpetual negative cycle that leads to an emotionally and biologically imbalanced Physical Center.

Stephen Covey, the author of *Seven Habits of Highly Effective People* talks about the benefits of the "Win-Win," meaning there are mutual benefits in a given situation. Incorporating exercise and increased physical activity into your daily life is a Win-Win-Win for you. First, you benefit physically of course. You see the results of your effort in decreased weight, increased muscle tone, the ability to wear smaller clothes, and seeing a more toned reflection in your mirror. Second, you benefit from a better attitude as your mindset and overall outlook improve with the increase in endorphins produced as you exercise (endorphins are your brain's natural painkillers that make you feel good). Third, you benefit from improved self esteem, the result of looking and feeling better. Win-Win-Win! Move it and lose it, as they say!

In the preceding paragraph, I noted both "exercise" and "increased physical activity." Perhaps you thought I was being redundant. Actually, the distinction between exercise and increased physical activity is important. You need to increase *both* following bariatric surgery.

Physical activity simply means movin' your groove thing. Getting your body in motion. Exercise, on the other hand, involves physical exertion, usually involving that nasty bodily function of sweating (I know you hate that), with the goal of burning calories and improving cardiovascular health.

Jot down the physical activities you do throughout your day. Things like:

- getting out of bed and moving about as you get ready for the day
- walking from the car to work or into the day care center or the grocery store or church or the mall

- walking to the mailbox
- going up or down any stairs in your home or office
- walking through the store, the school, the office hallways, and your home

Realistically, we have minimal physical activity in our adult lives unless we put effort into it. Admit it, whenever possible, you take elevators or escalators to go from floor to floor, and you use moving sidewalks if they are available. We spend a lot of time in our cars during a day, sometimes circling the parking lot waiting for the spot closest to our destination to become available. Many obese people simply choose to stay at home instead of putting forth the physical effort needed to go out.

"I used to stay home as much as possible," Rhonda said. "It was no fun to go anywhere if I had to walk any distance at all when I weighed over 300 pounds. I thought it was ridiculous when people at the support group suggested that doing 'the little things' like parking farther from the store or making an extra lap around the mall just to window shop would make any difference in how I felt. The truth is those things were my first form of 'exercise.' Without them, I don't know how I would have gotten into the habit of moving at all. Now I belong to the gym and love using the different machines there. I still do 'the little things' and encourage others who have just had bariatric surgery to do the same. They see me now at 143 pounds and it gives them hope that they, too, will be able to exercise and to enjoy it."

Think about exercising, moving your arms and legs, getting your heart rate up, sweating, feeling the burn! Think also about melting away pounds, decreasing your blood pressure and cholesterol, extinguishing diabetes, wearing smaller sizes, and smiling when you look in the mirror!

Let's do something with any unpleasant thoughts, feelings and memories of negative experiences you hold related to exercise. Imagine a jar with a lid. The lid is not on the jar, but you have the lid. Take a minute and allow yourself to think every negative thought you have about exercise. As you say each one to yourself, imagine it sliding into that jar. "I hate to sweat," you might say as you see those words just flowing into your jar and sitting at the bottom. Get them all in there. "Exercise is boring." "Exercising hurts." "I can't afford to go to the gym/purchase exercise gear and/or equipment." "I don't have time to exercise." "I don't see results fast enough." "I'm no good at sports or other forms of exercise." "People make fun of me when I exercise." "I'm too tired to exercise." "I don't feel like exercising." "It's not fun." "I hate it, I hate it, I hate it." When all of the negative thoughts are inside that imaginary jar, move on to your feelings related to exercise.

"I feel angry when I exercise." See those words fall into your jar. "I am embarrassed when I exercise." "I feel disgusted with myself because I don't exercise." "I am hurt because I was laughed at when I exercised." Now think of any negative experiences you personally had related to exercising. Maybe you kicked the soccer ball into the wrong team's goal. Perhaps you didn't fit into the PE uniforms in middle school. You may have been the person chosen last for team sports. Whatever your negative memories are, put them into that jar. When you have all the negative thoughts, feelings and memories in the jar, envision yourself putting the lid on the jar. Now find a shelf somewhere in your mind and set that closed jar on it. You may have to find it later… not to take any of those negatives back out but because you may remember other bad thoughts, feelings or experiences related to exercise that you'll need to add to the jar. Never fear – the jar can never be filled so you have no excuse to hold on to anything negative related to exercising. Any time in the future you find yourself complaining or moaning about exercising, think of this jar and mentally beam that negative thought or feeling into the jar on a shelf in your mind.

You *have to* exercise if you want to lose your weight and keep it off. I can't even pretend to sugarcoat this. There is no way around it, so let me say it again. If you want to lose weight and keep it off, you must exercise. For the rest of your life. Period. Now that we have established that fact, let's discuss what kind of exercise you want to do.

The choice is up to you, your sense of adventure, your creativity, and, of course, your current physical ability. There are fairly standard forms of exercise, which include: walking, jogging, swimming, playing tennis and bicycling. Many people enjoy rowing, martial arts, kickboxing, mountain biking, and hiking. Recently, belly dancing and other forms of aerobic dance have become popular forms of exercise. Roller skating, roller blading, ice skating, playing volleyball, playing basketball, engaging in yoga or Pilates, jumping rope and hula hooping can be exercise. Book stores and video stores have hundreds of exercise programs you can stretch with, dance to and tone with. They have fun titles like *Shrink Your Female Fat Zones* by Denise Austin, *Walk Away Your Waistline* by Leslie Sansone, and *Luscious - The Bellydance Workout for Beginners*, so they must be fun! Think how lucky you are to be able to watch these on your television screen in front of you. I was in my early 20's when Jane Fonda's first exercise album (as in vinyl) came out. I twisted and contorted myself in a hundred different ways trying to figure out what in the world she was describing while she went merrily along her way. "Stand with your feet a little more than hip distance apart, stomach pulled tight, buttocks pulled in…" "Flat back, straight legs, bounce, bounce, bounce, bounce…" I advanced to a VHS tape of *Kathy Smith's Fat-Burning Workout* tape six years later. My twin daughters were only four years old and they would dance along with Kathy and me in the living room. "Now add the knees… One, two, one, two, three…" "Kick it out…" "Shake it out, come on!" The girls still talk about that video and they are in their 20's! Which reminds me of another benefit of your exercising - you teach your children the value of doing so through your example. And remember – children learn what they live.

Choose exercise that fits your personality. "I had to get out of the house to exercise," Maury said. "Not only did I have to get out the house, I had to choose exercise that allowed me to be outdoors. The idea of going to a gym was stifling for me. I started out doing solitary exercise because I knew I wasn't fit enough to participate in group exercise. So I walked, first just in the neighborhood and then at the track behind the school. After I lost 40 pounds, I decided it would be more fun to exercise with other people. I'm a social guy and wanted to be around other people. I joined a local tennis league because when I was in high school I was a good tennis player. I have been playing on the league for the past six years. Now that I am at the healthy weight of 185 pounds and have built up good stamina, I am signing up for my first 5K run. I feel great and I have fun exercising."

Brandi was a homebody. She said, "I'm an introvert by nature. I have friends I see on a regular basis, but I like alone time and I love being home. I bought myself an elliptical machine. I was only able to use it for five minutes at a time when I got it. I weighed 215 pounds at that time and hadn't done any kind of exercise for years. Every week

I added another minute of time. As I lost weight it became easier and easier to work out on my elliptical. I now use it five times a week for 45 minutes each time. I warm up and cool down for 8 minutes before and after by doing a series of stretches. At 140 pounds, I love how I look and how I feel."

"I have Attention Deficit Disorder in everything I do," Stephen said. "That includes exercise. I get bored if I do the same thing over and over so I mix it up. Some days I go to the gym and do weight machines and the treadmill. Some days I run for an hour. Once in a while I join a pickup basketball game. I do what I feel like doing each day, but make sure I exercise every day. Annie Gottlier said in one of the *Chicken Soup for the Soul* books, 'It's so hard when I have to, and so easy when I want to.' Exercise doesn't feel like a 'have to' in my life any more like it did before my surgery."

Easier Said Than Done?

I worked in door-to-door encyclopedia sales before I went back to school to get my Ph.D. in Psychology. One of the sales strategies we were taught was the importance of "assuming the sale." This meant I was to proceed with my sales presentation assuming all along that the mom and dad I was working with were definitely going to buy the books. Likewise, I am assuming that you are buying the reality that you are going to exercise every day and that you're going to like it.

I hear your thoughts: "Right lady. It's easier said than done to get out there and exercise when you weigh what I weigh." "It's hard." "I don't have time." WAIT! We already went through all of those. There's no room for negative thoughts!

If you want to lose your weight and keep it off, you have to exercise. Period. In dealing with life after bariatric surgery, there can be no excuses. You must take personal responsibility for your choices and your actions. Choose to increase your physical activity. Choose to exercise regularly. Choose to enjoy it.

The Objections to Exercise

Just for fun (mine), let me review the list of objections to exercise, followed by a very direct, no-nonsense response. While the responses may 'sting', they are also true.

Objection to exercise: "I hate to sweat."
Response: You hate to sweat? How do you like taking insulin for diabetes and those five different medications for your high blood pressure and high cholesterol? Sweating means you are getting healthier and can very likely get rid of the insulin, the other meds, and many diseases. You choose. Sweat or continue with your diseases.

Objection to exercise: "Exercise is boring."
Response: Exercise can be boring. You have the choice of what kind of exercise you do. If you choose exercise that is boring to you, then it's no one's fault but your own that you're bored.

Objection to exercise: "Exercising hurts."
Response: Exercising may hurt. Without a doubt, *not* exercising has hurt you. Your obesity has led to a number of health problems that not only cause you physical pain, but are literally damaging your organs. With exercise, pain is gain. Without exercise, pain is eventually more pain.

Objection to exercise: "I can't afford to go to the gym/purchase exercise gear and/or equipment."
Response: You may not be able to go to the gym or purchase exercise equipment. Walking is free. Jogging is free. You need good shoes for these things? True. How much are you spending eating out each week? How much do your obesity-related medications cost? You CAN afford to exercise. In fact, can you afford not to?

Objection to exercise: "I don't have time to exercise."
Response: We make time for the things we want to make time for. What are your favorite television shows? How much time do you spend watching shows you could choose to give up in exchange for improved health via time spent exercising? How much time do you spend reading or talking on the phone or emailing? You *can* make time. Try recording your TV shows and watching them while you walk on the treadmill!

Objection to exercising: "I don't see results quickly enough."
Response: Is it better to see results slowly than not to exercise because you don't see results as quickly as you would like? Remember to employ logical thinking and get rid of stinkin' thinkin' (negative thoughts).

Objection to exercising: "I'm no good at sports or other forms of exercise."
Response: To get good at something you have to practice. Not only that, you don't *have* to be good at exercise to do it and receive the health benefits. You just have to do it.

Objection to exercising: "People make fun of me when I exercise."
Response: Not a problem. Exercise by yourself and be kind to yourself.

Objection to exercising: "I'm too tired to exercise/I don't feel like it."
Response: Give me a break! We're all too tired! And too busy. But we still do a lot of things. And it's widely known that when you exercise regularly, you have more energy!

Objection to exercising: "It's not fun."
Response: Fun! Make it fun or don't! That is your choice. Your mind set. You must exercise either way if you want what you say you want: sustained weight loss and better health.

Objection to exercising: "I hate it, I hate it, I hate it."
Response: Oh. See above response. (That is your choice. Your mind set. You must exercise either way if you want what you say you want: sustained weight loss and improved health.)

Sometimes the truth isn't soft and fluffy. Working with addictions, (chemical or behavioral), often requires direct, honest, no-nonsense responses.

"It Didn't Work"

Every week I spend one full day conducting pre-surgical interviews for people seeking bariatric surgery. Recently, I had an experience unlike any I have had in the past seven years doing those interviews. I don't schedule the appointments for the patients, so I have no idea who I will be seeing on any particular day. This day I looked at the schedule to see who my next patient was. The name I saw sounded familiar to me. When I saw the patient, I definitely recognized her. I greeted Wendy warmly, telling her I remembered meeting her several years ago when she had attended an information session for bariatric surgery. As far as I knew, she had already had surgery and I was confused as to why she was there. She was still quite heavy, and before I could ask, she blurted out why she was there. Wendy was very upset and said she was back at the bariatric center because her surgery "didn't work." I was taken off guard and asked her to please explain. She informed me that she had indeed had a bariatric procedure, had lost a great deal of weight, but in recent years she had put it back on. She was livid because her surgery "didn't work."

Unfortunately, Wendy's story is not uncommon enough. Many people regain a significant amount of the weight they initially lost following a bariatric procedure. I asked Wendy what she was eating, how often she was eating, if she was eating breakfast, if she was drinking a lot of water, how much exercise she was getting, if she was keeping a log of her food intake and her exercise, and if she was getting enough sleep. I was grateful when she admitted she was not following the eating guidelines as she had been instructed, nor was she exercising regularly. She was not keeping eating or exercise logs and rarely ate breakfast. Although she was upset and probably didn't want to hear it, the reality was that she had regained her weight because she was not doing what she had been instructed to do.

Gotta Do Ems Again

I mentioned in Chapter 3 that when I went to treatment for alcohol and drug dependency, I was told to do a few simple things and I did them, which helped me form the basis for my 20 years of sobriety (thank you, God). You now have a list of specific things you need to do to lose your weight and keep it off, your Gotta Do Ems (GDEs). Here they are again:

- make consistently healthy food choices (protein first)
- maintain portion control
- exercise on a regular basis (daily)
- drink plenty of water throughout the day, but not with meals
- eat breakfast
- plan your meals and follow your plan
- keep food and exercise journals
- get good rest

- utilize a healthy support system (support group meetings and on-line support)
- participate in individual and/or group counseling for at least a year

In losing weight and sustaining that weight loss, you must be direct and honest with yourself (do not permit excuses). You must focus on the present. Today is all you need to worry about. You don't need to lament over the fact that you "have to exercise every day of your life forever more." Simply focus on the fact that you are *choosing* to exercise *today.* Focus on what you can do today, thinking optimistically, and following through with realistic, specific goals: "I can think positively about my choice to exercise. I am grateful that I am healthy enough to exercise. Today I choose to exercise by walking two miles." No excuses. Exercising is a GDE.

Remember the importance of maintaining balanced Cognitive and Emotional Centers. Balance in those areas of life will assist you in balancing your Physical Center. Think positively about exercising and the benefits it holds for you. Make a list of the benefits of exercising on a regular basis. It can begin with the following:

- better mental attitude about health, looks, completing GDEs
- better emotional health – more optimism
- better physical health (decreases in diabetes, high blood pressure, high cholesterol, fewer body aches and pains)
- improved physical appearance
- increased energy

Exercise is an essential part of balancing your Physical Center. Healthy food choices are also vitally important.

You Are What You Eat

"You are what you eat" is not exactly a literal expression, but it's kind of funny to think about what the world would look like if that were true. If you looked like the thing you ate the most of, what would we see? For me, the picture would have changed over time. As a kid, I probably would have been an Oreo cookie. I could have rolled back and forth to school instead of having to walk every day. In high school, I would have been part chocolate shake and part cheese popcorn. Not a pretty sight, I think! In college… well, at first I would have been practically invisible since I ate almost nothing (and weighed nearly the same). Then I would have been liquid. Alcohol of one sort or another. Tragic. I'd have sloshed around campus and from one bar to another. During my first pregnancy, I would have been a waddling piece of peanut butter and jelly toast. As I lost the fifty pounds from the excess of PB&J after the birth of my son, I would have been a bowl of Total cereal – with lots and lots of milk. When I was pregnant with my twin daughters, I would have looked really funny. I'd have been half ham and sweet potatoes, and the other half cream cheese pineapple pie. Currently, I guess I would be part yogurt and part boneless, skinless chicken breast cooked in a Crockpot so that it falls apart at the touch of a fork… does that suggest I look flaky?

What a fun review of what I ate the most of at different times in my life! I've clearly gotten healthier this decade. But if I literally had to look like any of those foods, well, I simply couldn't choose! I think I'd want to look like something more colorful such as a vegetable medley. That sounds like the kind of healthy and pretty picture I'd like to portray!

As I think about it, the saying "You are what you eat" does have some almost-literal merit. Try the above exercise for yourself. Write down what you ate the most of over different periods of your life and think about what you looked like then. As I indicated above, when I went to college, I nearly quit eating and I looked like a person who rarely ate. My appearance was an outward acknowledgement of the sickness on the inside of me, both physically and emotionally. Anyone who is 5'4", 19 years old and weighs less than 90 pounds is either very physically or psychologically ill.

I mentioned that if I had looked like the alcohol that was my primary form of sustenance during the latter half of my college years, I'd have "sloshed" about campus. In truth, I'll bet that's how I appeared to others… sloshed, whether I was drunk or not.

If a person eats mostly foods that are high in fat, they are going to add additional fat to their body and will look fat. If they primarily eat foods that are lean, then they are going to look lean. Makes a lot of sense. *How do you want to look?*

Doctor's Orders

Following your bariatric procedure, it is essential that you eat the types of foods in portion sizes according to your doctor's guidelines. The dietary guidelines for post-bariatric surgery are well researched and have been refined with the assistance of people who have had the surgery. Everyone wants you to succeed. If you follow the instructions you are given related to what and how to eat following bariatric surgery, you will have few or no problems being able to tolerate food as your body heals.

There are too many variations in the specifics that one physician or nutritionist may recommend for me to outline postsurgical eating guidelines here. It is safe to say, however, that you will be directed to follow a progression from clear liquid to creamed soups to food the consistency of baby food to soft foods and finally the introduction of solid food. Please, for your own benefit, do what you are told! Follow this sequence for the recommended amount of time and only after each period of time ends should you move on to the next phase of food reintroduction. Also be sure to take your vitamins, drink plenty of water (except for 30 minutes before and after your meals), and eat protein first at every meal.

The Doctor Said I Could

My good friend Sally, who recently had the Gastric Sleeve procedure, helped me recognize that bariatric patients are given numerous mixed messages by the myriad of professionals they see before and after their procedures. The surgeon may say it's okay to eat something, whereas the nutritionist says it's not. Some nurses say it's all right to eat such-and-such while another says the same thing will cause all sorts of problems. Differing opinions from so many sources does, indeed, cause confusion.

My favorite example is a hot dog. Calvin showed me his post-surgical food diary. For the most part, he was eating foods that were nutritious and that followed the post-surgical guidelines the nutritionist had given him. I noticed, however, that he had hot dogs listed on his food diary four days of the week, so I asked him about that. "I love hot dogs," he replied with that unspoken "Yuuuummmmmy" in his tone. "Hot dogs," I said flatly, with that unspoken, "You've got to be kidding me" quality. Quickly and defensively, he countered, "The doctor said I could!" I questioned, "The doctor said you could have hot dogs?" "Yes, he did." Calvin replied defiantly. Now, using my softest, kindest, most therapeutic voice, I explained, "Calvin, I believe you when you say that the doctor said you can eat hot dogs. My reaction is not because you have eaten hot dogs. I am astounded that your surgeon, a medical doctor who is aware of your battle with food and weight, would tell you that it is okay to eat a hot dog or any other food that is so unhealthy. Did you know, Calvin, that one Hormel hot dog is 85% fat? Hot dogs aren't a healthy food choice for anyone, and especially not for a person who is working to lose weight and keep it off. After you have weight loss surgery, you need to eat foods that are nutritious and refrain from foods that are not good for you." With genuine interest and concern, Calvin asked, "Then why did the doctor say I could eat hot dogs?" I answered, "I can only guess that he was thinking in terms of whether or not your stomach could tolerate a hot dog, given that you had weight loss surgery. But Calvin, just because you can physically digest a hot dog, doesn't mean it is a good choice for you. Remember this: *If you want to be a virtuous person, you do the things virtuous people do. If you want to be an educated person, you do the things educated people do. If you want to be a healthy person with a healthy weight, you do the things a healthy person at a healthy weight does – eat right and exercise."*

It's What You're Eating and What's Eating You

Far too often post-bariatric patients end up back in the hospital or in tremendous pain because they decide to *do things their way* and eat foods they are not supposed to. Few things get my blood boiling more at the support group meetings than when I hear patients who have had the surgery telling those contemplating the surgery, "Yeah, I was eating whatever I wanted two weeks after my surgery." In my mind I'm thinking, "Yeah, and I'll probably see you a year and a half from now when you've gained back fifty pounds." If a person isn't willing to follow the instructions they were given for being healthy only two weeks after their surgery, it does not bode well for their long-term success.

Justin was 25 years young when he had gastric bypass surgery, and not quite past the adolescent stage of knowing more than those "old" middle-aged people at the support group meetings who were having surgery. "I knew plenty of people who had bariatric surgery. They all gave me advice about what to do after surgery, and so did the doctor and the nutritionist. I listened but guess I didn't pay that much attention. I figured because I was young that my body would be able to heal faster and handle things better than most of those people. I was 'good' for the first two or three weeks and then I started eating what I wanted when I wanted it. I got sick and threw up a couple of times so I stopped eating my old favorite foods for a while. I thought that if I just ate less of what I loved to eat, I would be just fine. I lost weight, of course because I couldn't physically eat as much as I did before the surgery. But, over three years, I gained back 85 of the 120 pounds I lost. I chose to go back to the support group, joined Weight Watchers and changed what and when I ate. I also got serious about exercise. Now, at age 30, standing six feet tall, I weigh 190 pounds. I look healthy and feel great. I definitely wish I had been less arrogant and more willing to listen to those who truly knew better than me. What I ate and how often I ate led me to gain back my weight."

For Larissa, it was what she was eating and what was eating her that resulted in a weight regain of 67 pounds two years after losing 105 pounds. "I was working for the Department of Family and Children's Services when I had my surgery. My job was to investigate reports of child abuse and to remove kids from their homes, if necessary. After my surgery, I did what the doctor and nutritionist said for the first eight or nine months. My weight fell off and I was looking and feeling good. I attended the support group meetings regularly and spent a lot of time on the Internet web sites for bariatric patients. My life pretty much revolved around losing weight at that time. I'm a single woman so it was easy for me to devote a lot of attention to my weight loss. Almost a year after I had surgery, I was assigned a case at work which led to tremendous emotional disruption in my life. I was sent to investigate what I assumed was another 'average' abuse case. Although none of the situations in which a child is abused or neglected is easy for me, I had become somewhat desensitized over the years. This case, however, triggered memories of my own abuse. I had buried the memories so deeply I had completely forgotten about them.

For work I was sent to the home of a child who had been intentionally burned by her mother's boyfriend. I had seen cigarette burns on children hundreds of time, which was what I was expecting in this situation.

What I saw on this two-year old boy were feet with third degree burns covering half of those teeny, tiny feet. My initial reaction, I thought, was due to the physical horror of the actual burns. Fortunately, I was able to perform my job duties and got medical help for the child. The investigation itself took several weeks. Over the course of the investigation, I found myself uncharacteristically eating foods I hadn't had since before my bariatric procedure. I started going to Dairy Queen! The place I vowed never to set foot in again. I isolated myself from friends I had met at the weight loss support group and made excuses to skip the meetings. I stayed off the Internet and made no attempts to talk to anyone about the negative behavior changes I was making. My behavior didn't even make sense to me but I didn't slow down and examine my thoughts. Instead, I slipped, almost unconsciously, into old, unhealthy eating patterns. I stopped exercising and became increasingly depressed. No one at work said anything to me about my increasing weight. The downward cycle might not have stopped if I hadn't developed a terrible case of bronchitis, which sent me to my primary care physician. She knew me well, although I hadn't been to see her for almost a year. I made an appointment when I came down with bronchitis. One look at me and she began asking questions. 'Are you going to the support group meetings? Are you exercising regularly? Are you maintaining eating and exercise diaries? How are things with your parents and siblings? Are you in a relationship? How is your sleep?' On and on she went with the questions. Because I trusted this woman, I told the truth. She recognized that I was clinically depressed and, in spite of my initial objections, informed me that she was arranging an appointment for me to see a psychotherapist. I agreed to go, and although I tried to convince myself to cancel the session, I went. In the first two sessions, the therapist was able to help me pinpoint when I changed my good eating and exercise habits. She assisted me in figuring out what was going on in my life at that time. I found myself talking about the little boy with the burned feet and how it upset me more than most of the cases I see. The therapist noted a change in my tone of voice when I spoke about this. During the next few weeks, I remembered that I, too, had been badly burned on the feet in an act of child abuse. The therapist helped me see that the trauma of seeing that burned child on my job had unleashed deeply buried memories of my own abuse.

I was using food in an attempt to ward off the painful emotions that were trying to surface. With the help of the therapist, the support of my friends from the bariatric support group, a lot of soul-searching, crying, journaling, and self-love, I was able to address the issues related to the abuse. I also started eating right again, began exercising and lost almost all of the weight I had regained. I still go to therapy now and then. I always go to the support group meetings and I encourage other people who are having weight loss surgery to seek professional help. They may not even know they need it! For me, gaining my weight back after I had lost it was a result of what I was eating AND what was eating me. I had to deal with both to get healthy."

What you have been eating and what's been eating you led to your obesity. Being obese, in turn, directly affected your self image and your body image.

What Do You See When You Look in the Mirror?

The National Eating Disorders Association (NEDA) describes body image as how people see themselves when they look in the mirror or in their mind, what people believe about their own appearance, how they feel about their bodies, and how they sense and control their bodies as they move. The NEDA says that people with a negative body image have a distorted perception of their shape, feel ashamed, feel self-conscious, are anxious about their body, feel uncomfortable in their body, and are convinced that only other people are attractive. The organization also notes that people with negative body image have a greater likelihood of developing an eating disorder and are more likely to suffer from feelings of depression, isolation, low self-esteem, and to be obsessed with weight loss.

On the other hand, the group describes persons with a positive body image as having a true perception of their natural shape and understanding that physical appearance says very little about character and value as a person. People with a positive body image do not spend an unreasonable amount of time worrying about food, weight, and calories. They feel comfortable and confident in their body.

On its website (www.NationalEatingDisorders.org) NEDA states: "We all may have our days when we feel awkward or uncomfortable in our bodies, but the key to developing positive body image is to recognize

107

and respect our natural shape and learn to overpower those negative thoughts and feelings with positive, affirming, and accepting ones." That sounds like it could have come straight from the previous chapter, with its focus on replacing negative thoughts with positive thoughts, which leads to positive feelings and behaviors. Balancing your Cognitive, Emotional, and Physical Centers is hard work, but with practice, you can do this – if you choose to. Your health is your responsibility!

My Head is Spinnin'

Are you old enough to remember the song *Dizzy* by Tommy Roe? The lyrics in the chorus are, "I'm so dizzy, my head is spinnin'. Like a whirlpool, it never ends." During the first several months following bariatric surgery your body changes at an amazing pace. You lose weight very rapidly, people comment frequently and enthusiastically about how good you look, you feel better, and your perceptions about yourself, other people, and the world change. Your physical body changes much more quickly than your mental image of your body.

Listening to patients talk about body image, before and after surgery, is interesting, to say the least. A fair number of obese people report feeling "shocked," "amazed," and "confused" when they see pictures of themselves. "Even though I knew what the number on the scale was," Sandy reported, "I didn't think of myself as being fat. Every time I saw pictures of myself, I was aghast. I was able to see how large I really was in the photos, but when I looked in a mirror, I never saw that fat person. I know I will have to work on the mental body image as I continue to lose weight. I can't afford to remain 'blind' to how I see myself in real life or I risk gaining my weight back."

Alice said, "I knew I was fat. I felt fat, and the scale confirmed that I was fat. I saw fat when I looked in the mirror. However, when I looked at pictures of myself, I didn't see a fat person. The truth is I rarely looked at myself in pictures. If I didn't look at myself, I didn't have to acknowledge how big I really was. I didn't want to see it because the reality would only further depress me. I already felt horrible about myself. Seeing pictures of me at such a heavy weight would have added to my already miserable body image."

Maria told me, "Even though I lost 170 pounds after surgery and got down to 138 pounds, I still thought of myself as a fat person. I continued to feel fat and told myself my body was still ugly. I remained very self-conscious about my weight and shape. It seemed like I had gone through the surgery and all the work it took to lose the weight only to remain ashamed of how I looked. I sort of gave up and fell into the 'why bother' mindset. I re-gained 35 pounds and thankfully, got into therapy. It has been hard work, but well worth it. I'm back down to 145 pounds. In spite of occasionally wishing my thighs were smaller or my stomach tighter, I like my body. The positive changes in my body image are starting to catch up with the positive changes resulting from my weight loss."

The Dressing Room Surprise

"I was able to buy the dress for my daughter's wedding three sizes smaller than I expected!" "For the first time since I was a teenager, I was able to fit into clothes at the trendy stores!" "Never will I have to buy 'Husky' clothes again." Comments like these from surgical weight-loss patients are exhilarating. Smiles and tears of joy are shared by men and women experiencing the rewards of their hard efforts to follow the guidelines for weight loss following surgery. Sometimes, along with the thrills associated with weight loss, come surprising, painful emotions.

Brenda found herself staring in the mirror at the clothing store where she had always wanted to shop. "Before I had my surgery, I wrote out a goal: 'To buy clothes at the quaint little boutique downtown.' For years I would pass by there on my way to work and stare into the windows admiring the clothes. I knew I couldn't fit into anything in the store so I never went in. But I dreamed on and on after surgery about going into the boutique and trying on every adorable outfit I saw and buying whatever I wanted! As soon as I knew I could fit into something, anything, in the store, I went. All by myself. Shopping at the boutique was a dream I had kept to myself, and I wanted to celebrate it as a personal accomplishment.

"I held my breath as I entered the store," Brenda continued. "I took in every sight and smell. I took my time and admired clothing on every single rack. I carefully chose four outfits to have the sales clerk take to the dressing room. I walked into the dressing room beaming with pride and satisfaction. I took the first garment off the hanger with the care you take when holding a newborn baby. It was a lilac blouse, made of pure silk. It felt so soft and delicate on my hand. I carefully put my arms into the sleeves and buttoned it. It was a "Large." It fit!

"I waited to look in the mirror until after I had put on the light grey slacks I had chosen to go with the blouse. A size 14. Would they fit? I'm sure I held my breath as I put each leg into the pants and gently pulled up the zipper. To my tremendous joy and satisfaction, they zipped up easily. I let myself breathe and finally risked a peek in the mirror. To my disbelief, there were tears rolling down my cheeks as I saw this vision of loveliness staring back at me from the dressing room mirror!

"I wondered about my tears. I couldn't get them to stop. I just stood there and wept. This wasn't what I had expected. In all my anticipation and daydreaming of the trip to the boutique, there had been no weeping! These were not tears of joy, which I could have understood. Sadness oozed from every pore of my being. I have no idea how long I stayed in the dressing room crying. I didn't try on the other outfits that day. I composed myself as well as I could, although there was no hiding the fact that I had just completely melted down in the dressing room. As badly as I wanted to leave the store unnoticed, I was not going without purchasing that size 14 slacks and the Large silk, lilac blouse. The clerk very kindly said nothing about my tear-stained face, but wrapped up my purchases with care.

"I went straight home and began to write," Brenda remembered. "With no effort, out poured the thoughts and feelings those tears represented. The years of longing to wear such lovely clothing in smaller sizes appeared in words on my notepad. The sadness of seeing others walking out of the boutique and never thinking it would be me walking out of there with a package of clothing for myself revealed itself. I grieved. I ached to my soul. I wrote for a very long time. When the words stopped appearing, I made a conscious decision to wrap up my discourse with positive words. I wrote: 'Today's tears were filled with unspoken thoughts and feelings related to the past. They were the visual representation of healing for my body and spirit. I am grateful for the experience of going to the boutique, delighting in the sensory experience of the store itself, for the kindness of the sales clerk, and definitely for my stunning new outfit. I am grateful for the hard work and effort I have put into my recovery from obesity, including the healthy eating choices, the exercise and the support I get from my friends. I look forward to future shopping adventures and will accept whatever thoughts and emotions surface during them. I will continue to learn about myself as my healing journey continues.'"

When Conrad went into the dressing room of a store in which he longed to shop to try on his new, smaller size, he found himself feeling intensely angry. "It was alarming to me. I thought I was going to be proud and excited to fit into the cool clothes other young guys wear. When I saw myself in the mirror of the dressing room wearing these clothes I heard voices inside my head. The voices were shouting insults. I heard kids from elementary school calling me 'tub of lard.' I heard my baseball coach saying, 'If you don't lose some of that weight, boy, you won't be able to get yourself to first base without passing out.' I heard my dad back up the coach: 'He's right, Conrad. You'll look like a fool out there waddling to first base.' Worst of all, I heard my own voice: 'You fat pig. I hate you. You look like a sumo wrestler and you're not even 20 years old.' I had to get out of that store as fast as I could. I didn't buy one thing. It was several months and many therapy sessions later before I went back to that store."

In therapy, Conrad was able to work through his anger toward people who were mean to him when he was fat. He learned to forgive them and himself. He was able to build respect for himself because he continued to do the work it takes to be able to fit into the clothes he wanted so badly to wear.

Katie's trip to the dressing room unexpectedly led to a weight regain of 35 pounds. "I waited until I was at what I considered to be my ideal weight before I would allow myself to go shopping at the store of my dreams. I was a size 10, which I hadn't been since the 8th grade. I took a ton of clothes into the dressing room, and I bought almost everything I tried on. But I noticed that while I was in the dressing room, I felt a bit short of breath and seemed to be shaking a little. I remember having trouble with the buttons and zippers because my hands were unsteady. I felt almost like I was going to have a panic attack. During the next couple of weeks I wore every one of those awesome outfits I bought. I felt good in them but was also aware that I felt uncomfortable at the same time. Without even realizing it, I started eating more of the foods I had given up after surgery. It wasn't long before all my cute new clothes were too tight. I ignored my feelings about this and simply rearranged my closet like I have done hundreds of times in the past, based on what size clothing fit me at the present time."

With her therapist, Katie eventually figured out that she feared the attention that came with her new, form-fitting clothes. In the past, when Katie had lost weight, she had become extremely promiscuous. In therapy, she was able to realize that she could be at a healthy weight, look attractive, dress in fun clothes, and choose not to be promiscuous. Back down to a size 10, Katie said, "I like the way I look and the way I feel. I even like the way people look at me and compliment me. I love my new life and intend to keep it this way!"

Whether alone in a dressing room or receiving attention from others about the way you look, every person will have unique reactions to his or her new physical appearance. Unexpected emotions may arise as your body changes. You will likely need the help of friends or professionals to help you process the thoughts and feelings you experience related to your body image during these times of change. Your Physical Center is deeply intertwined with your Cognitive and Emotional centers.

Gotta Do Ems for a Balanced Physical Center

Maintaining balance in the Physical Center, as you have just read, requires you to assess and alter your body image. Balance in this center will be much easier if you do two of the most important Gotta Do Ems: maintain a food diary and maintain an exercise diary. These diaries are essential to sustaining your weight loss. Whether you like to, want to, or feel like it, MAINTAIN FOOD AND EXERCISE DIARIES IN ORDER TO SUSTAIN YOUR WEIGHT LOSS! I don't think I can adequately express in words the importance of doing this.

Keeping accurate food and exercise diaries helps you make sense of weight gains or losses. Let's say Mary loses 130 pounds in 14 months following surgery. She maintains both food and exercise logs. After her body settles into a healthy weight of 145 pounds, her weight remains steady most of the time. If she gains five or 10 pounds, Mary looks at her food and exercise charts to discover the reason for her weight gain. Maybe she has been eating at restaurants more often; perhaps she has been eating larger portions; she may have cut down on the number of times she exercises during the week, or some combination of these factors. Her food and exercise diaries help her determine what changes she has made which have resulted in her weight gain. She can therefore alter her behavior and bring her weight back to her 'new normal.'

Some fluctuation in weight is to be expected. In fact, many surgical weight loss patients will regain five to 10 percent of the weight they initially lose following surgery. In addition, physiological factors, such as menstrual cycles or water retention, can change your weight by a few pounds. However, if you find yourself steadily re-gaining weight, especially after keeping it steady for a period of time, it is almost certain you have engaged in one or more unhealthy behaviors.

Keeping eating and exercise logs helps you remain accountable for the choices you are making regarding:

- food selection
- the amount of food you eat
- your pattern of eating (frequency, time, location)
- how you feel when you eat
- the types of food you choose to eat
- the frequency with which you exercise
- the amount of time you exercise
- the type of exercise you choose

Why would a person *not* do such a simple thing as keep food and exercise diaries? Because they don't want to know/take responsibility for the choices they are making.

A recent pre-surgical interview with a 22-year-old female named Claressa illustrates the powerful effects of denial in regard to what one eats. Claressa said she and her fiancé broke off their engagement seven months before our interview. She explained that he had been unfaithful to her several times during their courtship and engagement. She always managed to make excuses for his behavior or said she believed him when he told her he had been faithful to her. One day she sat him down and asked him to be honest with her about what had been taking place with other women throughout their relationship. He finally, candidly shared the reality of his many trysts. In retrospect, Claressa was able to see how she kept herself from seeing the truth. Just as she allowed herself to deny the truth about her boyfriend cheating on her, she also denied the truth about how much she ate.

Maintaining a food diary is the most accurate way to remain completely honest about the types and quantities of food you eat as well as the frequency of your eating. I'm not talking about counting calories. The simplest type of food diary is nothing more than a list of what you ate during the day. A more useful food journal includes the amount of food you ate and when you ate it. A really *great* food journal would include:

- what you ate
- when you ate it
- the amount of food you consumed
- how you felt at the time you were eating

The easiest way I have found to keep a food log is on the "notes" section of my cell phone. I simply make a note that says, "January Food," put in the date and then makes entries such as: 1/6 – whole wheat toast, egg at 8:30 – in a hurry, excited for day; yogurt and egg white at noon – in a hurry, relatively relaxed; protein bar at 3:00 – relaxed, happy; chicken breast and cottage cheese at 6:00 – irritated; protein pudding at 8:30 – tired." Some people keep their food diaries on the computer. There are several Internet sites with wonderful food diaries, such as fitday.com, thedailyplate.com, and myfooddiary.com. Other people maintain a three ring binder with daily food and exercise journals combined. Make your food diary as simple or elaborate as you would like it to be. But do it. It's a GDE.

The same is true of your exercise diary. If you log what you do, you will be able to correlate your weight losses or increases to the reality of your food intake and exercise output.

Food and exercise diaries are about accountability. You are accountable for what you put into your mouth. You are responsible for writing it down. You are responsible for the type and amount of exercise you do. All of us want to avoid responsibility at one time or another, but if you want to lose weight and keep it off for a lifetime, you *must* be responsible for what you eat, how much you eat, how often you eat, and the exercise you do. It's your health and your responsibility to maintain it!

Weighing In

"I weigh myself every day." "I never weigh myself; I judge my weight by how my clothes feel." "I get on the scale once a week." "Once a month." How often should you weigh yourself? This is a tough question because there is not one answer that fits all.

Some people insist on weighing themselves every day. Honestly, I believe there are more dangers associated with this practice than there are benefits. To begin with, if it's true, as I am told by the vast majority of people during their pre-surgical interview, that the primary goal of losing weight is for health reasons, then weighing yourself daily should not be necessary. As noted earlier in the chapter, a person's weight is going to fluctuate within a few pounds day to day. If you see that you have gained a pound one day, it is not a reason for hysterics and yet, a person who weighs daily often becomes hysterical due to the increase of a single pound.

Seeing a number on a scale and allowing that number to ruin your mood for an hour or an entire day is a warning flag. For a number to have that kind of power over your emotions, and more importantly, over your sense of self, is an indication that there is a psychological issue present. When I was actively anorexic, I allowed the number on the scale to determine my worth as a human being. If the number on that scale increased even one pound, my sense of worth plummeted. Clearly, not healthy. I had to learn to refrain from weighing myself until I was able to fully accept that my sense of self worth was not to be determined by my numerical weight. To this day, I choose not to weigh myself very often. I eat healthy, I exercise regularly, I keep both food and exercise logs and my body has settled into a healthy weight for itself. The number on the scale isn't important.

Some people simply cannot be convinced not to weigh themselves every day. If weighing yourself daily works for you, then all right. Be aware, however, this compulsive behavior may indicate that "the number" on the scale has a wee bit too much influence in your life.

The purpose of you weighing yourself should be to keep track of the direction in which your weight is going. After your body loses its excess weight and settles into a healthy weight for you, the reason to get on the scale is to see that you are staying at a fairly steady weight. For some people, that will mean weighing themselves weekly, for others it may be every other week or monthly. Again, the purpose is to look for any major fluctuations or directional changes in weight. I recommend that people keep a visual graph of their weight, beginning with their weight at the time of surgery. Then, every week or month, record the date and your weight on the graph. The first year to two years after surgery, the bar on the graph decreases as your weight decreases. After your weight has stabilized, the graph will remain constant. If, at some point, the number on the scale begins to increase and an upward pattern develops, you should be able to look at your food and exercise diaries and see the reason why. If your weight is increasing steadily, and you have been diligent about filling out your food and exercise diaries honestly, then you should find an answer as to why your weight has been increasing in one or the combination of the diaries. If not, then you need to see your physician.

But I'm Hungry

How do you know when you're hungry? *Do* you know when you're hungry? What does physical hunger feel like in your body? The answer to that question will be different for different people. The physiological symptoms of genuine physical hunger include: headaches, feeling light-headed and/or weak, hearing or feeling your stomach rumble, feeling physically ill, sweating, and an empty, sometimes painful feeling in your stomach. Some people become irritable and may become nervous. True physical hunger is the connection between the brain and the rest of the body and its need for fuel. When we are genuinely, physically hungry we eat to give our bodies the energy and nutrition they need to function properly. If you wait to eat until you are extremely physically hungry, it is easy to overeat. You may be eating so quickly that you ingest more food than is healthy before your brain and stomach have made the connection that you are full. Eating quickly results in your eating more than your body needs. And then you feel full, stuffed, uncomfortable and probably remorseful.

Obese people often forget what it feels like physically to be reasonably full, the point at which you should stop eating. If you are obese, you have probably come to expect to feel stuffed before you stop eating. Feeling stuffed becomes the norm. It may be the case that you also have forgotten what physical hunger feels like. While there are some medical reasons a person may not experience normal physiological hunger and fullness signals, if you eat frequently or 'graze,' your body likely hasn't felt physical hunger for some time. Or, if you have ignored your body's hunger cues, you may have forgotten what they indicate.

Head Hunger Revisited

In Chapter 4, Mark and Kristy described what "head hunger" was to them. An emotional hunger, often related to habits and/or past circumstances, head hunger is often more of a problem for postsurgical weight-loss patients than physical hunger. Ann Capper, a registered dietician for FINDING balance, a faith-based nonprofit organization dedicated to helping those who struggle with eating and body image issues, refers to various "false alarm signals that are often confused with stomach hunger." As Capper writes, "They are legitimate sensations, but not true stomach hunger." She describes a number of examples of what I call head hunger -- for example, "teeth hunger," when "we want to chew our frustrations away" or "mouth hunger," when "we see or smell something that looks so delicious that our mouths start to water [and] we desire to taste the food, but really aren't physically hungry." Capper also describes "mind hunger," when we eat because the clock says it's time to do so, and "heart hunger," when we eat to fill an emotional ache or void. Being bored and being tired can also stimulate us to eat.

Whenever you feel hunger, it is always a good idea to ask yourself, "What, besides food, do I want or need right now?" Your Physical Center encompasses more than what you put in your mouth and exercise. Just as with your Cognitive and Emotional Centers, establishing balance in your Physical Center highlights your need for the support of other people as you make the choices and changes that lead to sustained weight loss. A healthy, balanced Social Center is integral to achieve your goal of a full, balanced life following bariatric surgery.

Chapter 5: End of Chapter Exercises

Balance Brainwork

    1) Make a list of all of the physical activities/forms of exercise you participated in during childhood, along with a few sentences about how much you did or did not enjoy each.

    2) Have an "out loud talk" to "Exercise" or write a letter beginning "Dear Exercise" and tell it (Exercise) what you like and don't like about it. Before you finish the talk or letter, decide that you are going to participate in exercise, whether you "like it" or not, and write that or say it out loud!

Balance Busters

Replace the following negative statements about exercise with positive statements that will lead to positive behavior.

Example:

Negative statement: "I hate to exercise/sweat." Positive replacement statement: "When I exercise and sweat, even though it is not my favorite thing to do, I know I am losing weight and getting healthier, which are my long-term goals, so I will keep right on exercising and sweating."

Negative statement: "I don't have time to exercise." Your positive replacement statement: _____

_____.

Negative statement: "It costs too much money to buy a gym membership, exercise equipment, and workout clothing." Your positive replacement statement: _____

_____.

Negative statement: "It hurts too much to exercise." Your positive replacement statement: _____

_____.

Balance Boosters

1) Make a list of all of the forms of physical activity/exercise that you have not participated in but think you would like to try. Be creative! Have you ever wanted to take dance lessons? Kick-boxing? Ice skating? If you have children or grandchildren, include activities they can participate in with you. Think of playing with them and getting the benefit of physical activity as well!

2) Make a weekly schedule of the exact times you will exercise, as well as the type of exercise you will do.

3) Get an exercise "coach." This can be a good friend (if he or she is a person who is willing to hold you accountable), a personal trainer, or a Life Coach who can help you stay focused on your goals, who will encourage you and will help you remain on task. Write down who you will choose as your exercise coach: _____

_____.

The Best of the Best

- "The *I* in illness is isolation, and the crucial letters in wellness are *we*." - Author unknown, as quoted in Mimi Guarneri, *The Heart Speaks: A Cardiologist Reveals the Secret Language of Healing*

- "The greatest wealth is health." - Virgil

- "Health is a state of complete physical, mental and social well-being, and not merely the absence of disease or infirmity." - World Health Organization, 1948

- "In order to change we must be sick and tired of being sick and tired." - Author Unknown

- "If you have health, you probably will be happy, and if you have health and happiness, you have all the wealth you need, even if it is not all you want." - Elbert Hubbard

- "The longer I live the less confidence I have in drugs and the greater is my confidence in the regulation and administration of diet and regimen." - John Redman Coxe, 1800

- "When it comes to eating right and exercising, there is no 'I'll start tomorrow.' Tomorrow is disease." - V.L. Allineare

- "If you don't take care of yourself, the undertaker will overtake that responsibility for you." - Carrie Latet
- "Doctors are always working to preserve our health and cooks to destroy it, but the latter are the more often successful." - Denis Diderot
- "He who has health has hope; and he who has hope has everything". -Arabic Proverb
- "A bodily disease, which we look upon as whole and entire within itself, may, after all, be but a symptom of some ailment in the spiritual part." - Nathaniel Hawthorne, *The Scarlet Letter*

Cardinal Convictions

Write three Cardinal Convictions you will make part of your daily self-talk to remind yourself that participating in regular physical exercise is essential to your long term goal of sustained weight loss. For example: "Exercising is a choice I make every day that helps me feel better physically and emotionally!"

Write this reminder everywhere you need to in order to keep it in mind at all time:

My Heatlh. My Responsibility. This Day. Every Day.

CHAPTER 6

Do I Know You?-- Your Social Center

"A healthy social life is found only, when in the mirror of each soul the whole community finds its reflection, and when in the whole community the virtue of each one is living."

-- *Rudolf Steiner*

Who Am I?

"Who am I?" is a question that has intrigued humans for as long as we have been on this planet. That question, "Who am I?" looms in the minds of surgical weight-loss patients as they shed pounds, inches, and clothing sizes. Obese people travel up and down the scale trail many times. The thin self is often described as being more confident, outgoing, and much more physically and socially active. The heavy self is described as one who stays home, fears being around people, has little energy, and spends very little time or effort on physical endeavors or at social events. In short, the obese person does not like being seen by others. Being obese throws your Social Center seriously out of balance.

Is it actually your weight that determines how involved you choose to be with others? Objectively speaking, you were probably less socially active when you were heaviest. Yet, it's not really your BMI that dictates how social you may be. Think back to Chapter 4 and recall that your thoughts about yourself and your beliefs about what others think of you may well have led to your socially isolating behavior.

"When I'm fat, I criticize myself and feel badly about myself," said

Michael, a long-time weight yo-yo'er. "I don't want to be around other people in social settings when I am at my heaviest. I compare myself to the thin people and know they are doing the same thing... thinking and feeling negatively about me. To avoid going through that, I stay home almost all the time when I'm in a 'fat phase.'"

The Other End of the Spectrum

Jillian tearfully shared her fears of becoming thin with her group members. "I'm scared to lose weight," she said. "I've done it before and when I'm thin I tend to have sex with a lot of different men. That leaves me feeling just as badly about myself as when I'm really fat." Rodney said when he loses a lot of weight, he engages in extramarital sexual activities "because I feel desired by women." Trina said she slept with a lot of different people whether she was fat or thin "because either way, I really wanted to feel like I was cared about. I hated myself all the time. I don't really believe in casual sex but I engaged in a lot of it." Gretchen said that when she lost weight in the past, she wanted to "go out and do things with the girls like shop, go to the movies, or meet for coffee. It's not that I'm doing anything that goes against my morals, but I neglect my husband and kids because I become overly involved in my social life and then I feel badly about that."

These patients are describing the socially-related psychological issues underlying their food and weight problems. After their weight-loss surgeries, Jillian and Rodney became aware of, and addressed, their need to be physically desired. As therapy progressed, they became aware that the need they were seeking to fill was more about being acknowledged and appreciated for who they were, and they learned to choose how to get that need met in healthy ways. Gretchen's needs were similar to those of Jillian and Rodney. Gretchen long to be acknowledged and appreciated -- by people other than her husband and children--but she met those needs through continual social interaction with friends. She did not understand the need for setting personal boundaries with others, nor did she recognize what her underlying needs were. Therefore, her Social Center became seriously imbalanced. Gretchen was spending too much time with friends and not enough time with family.

Staying home when one is overweight is one end of the unbalanced Social Center spectrum. The other end of the spectrum is engaging in social behaviors that go against personal values or spending too much time participating in social activities. A balanced Social Center lies somewhere in the middle: getting social needs met in healthy amounts and in healthy ways.

Personal Boundaries and Your Social Life

Personal boundaries. You hear a lot of talk about these things called "personal boundaries" in the world of therapy. What are they, anyway? And what do boundaries have to do with obesity and with your social life?

The word boundary suggests an edge or a line. Think about "a line drawn in the sand." If you're playing volleyball on a beach and you draw an out-of-bounds line in the sand, any play beyond that line does not count toward earning points. If you own property in a suburb and have neighbors on both sides of your home, you may install a privacy fence. The fence indicates where the boundaries of your property lie. Your neighbors are not permitted inside of these boundaries without your permission. "Personal boundaries" are invisible lines you draw that indicate how close, either physically or emotionally, you allow other people to get to you.

When you talk with a co-worker in the hall, you each maintain "personal space" without giving it much thought. If that co-worker stands too close to you during the conversation, you feel uncomfortable and probably back up. Your backing up is a way to establish a comfortable physical personal boundary. Let's say you don't know this co-worker very well. All previous conversations with them have been limited to work-related issues with perhaps a comment or two about a local sporting event or concert coming to town. Let's pretend that co-worker suddenly says to you in the midst of one of your typical work-related, in-the-hall chats, "So, how many sexual partners have you had?" After you pick your jaw up off the floor, you will be acutely aware of the personal discomfort elicited by such a personal (and inappropriate) question. That person has invaded your emotional "personal space" by asking that question. A person who has no personal boundaries of their own might respond with, "Well, now. Let me think for a just a moment. First there was.... Next it was... ." A person with healthier personal boundaries knows that a question about sexual partners by a co-

123

worker is completely inappropriate. The person with healthy personal boundaries would say something along the lines of, "I'm uncomfortable with that question. My personal matters are not something I discuss with acquaintances at my place of employment." This answer places a healthy boundary between you and that person.

People often discuss personal boundaries using the example of a fence. For example, a fence built around a house that has no gate for entry or exit is an example of boundaries that are too rigid. No one can enter or leave that yard. When a person is in a "fat phase" they tend to implement such boundaries. They stay home, spending as much time as possible there, interacting with as few people as possible. Margaret described having closed emotional boundaries with her husband, which became worse as she gained weight. "I completely shut him out of my world. In the evenings, we were in separate rooms watching different television shows. We slept in separate beds. I even stopped having meals with him. He tried to communicate with me. I was too self-absorbed. I loathed my weight and did not want to interact with anyone, not even my husband." Margaret's boundaries were closed.

If there is no fence around a house, anyone is free to come and go from the property at will. Jillian, Rodney and Gretchen were displaying a lack of boundaries by sleeping with random people and by spending too much time away from home when they were "skinny."

A house that has a fence with a gate at the front and back demonstrates healthy boundaries. People can come and go, but they must use the gates. As owner of the house, you can put locks on the gates at times if you choose. A healthy person, regardless of their weight, wants to have the equivalent of a fence with gates as their personal boundaries. They spend balanced amounts of time with friends, with family and by themselves.

Terri, a young adult, 5'3" tall, weighing 380 pounds described herself as "the fat girl in school." During her pre-surgical interview, I asked about her friendships throughout life. "I had friends," she said, "because I always did things for people. They took advantage of me." I asked what sorts of things she did for people. "If someone needed a ride home in high school, I always took them home. If people needed notes for a test, I gave them my notes. I gave people change for the soda machine if they needed it. I even wrote papers for people sometimes."

She readily acknowledged that she did these things to be "liked," fearing peers would reject her otherwise due to her weight. Terri did not set personal boundaries with people in an attempt to avoid rejection from them. She had no fence around her property. She did not say "no" to people.

A person with rigid boundaries (a fence with no gates) would never give a person in need a ride home, would never lend change for a soda, and would not share class notes, much less do another person's homework for them. Rob had rigid boundaries. "It wasn't because I was mean that I didn't offer to help others. I was fat and didn't want to risk being teased so I kept completely to myself. It was how I protected myself. To others, I guess I seemed rude." Rob didn't want to be hurt by anyone so he maintained rigid social boundaries, not allowing anyone to get close to him.

A person with healthy boundaries (a fence with gates) would give a person a ride home once in a while if doing so did not interfere with their own schedule. They would lend people change for a soda now and then, especially if they got paid back when they did so. They would give class notes to a person who had a legitimate reason for missing school. They would refuse to write a paper for a classmate, noting that doing so would be unhealthy for both of them. People with healthy boundaries open and shut the "gates" appropriately, according to the situation.

Healthy Emotional Boundaries

Either end of a continuum is usually not the balanced, or healthy place to be. Do you remember playing on a teeter-totter as a kid? Did you and the person on the other end try to balance the board so you were both off the ground and the board was balanced? Sometimes one or the other person had to scoot forward or back on their end of the teeter-totter to even up the weight distribution so it would balance. A balanced teeter-totter represents having good personal boundaries. Balancing the teeter-totter requires shifting forward or back a bit. So it is in life. To have a balance social life, you must make adjustments according to the different people in your life, your needs, their needs, your time demands, their time demands, and a host of other factors. Healthy personal boundaries are essential to having a healthy, balanced Social Center. Obese people very often have poor personal boundaries. Obese people often have imbalanced social lives.

If you are being taken advantage of (always the person offering to give rides or lend money for the soda machine), you need to adjust your behavior to develop healthier personal boundaries. If you have become the school's quarter-and-dime-money-machine, you probably feel angry, the result of being used by others. Many people who put themselves in situations where they feel used, see themselves as victims, although they have usually created the situation themselves. Mark was this guy. "Somehow, word got around that I always lent people change to buy a soda during lunch. I started making sure I had a bunch of change in my pockets before I went to school in the morning. After a while, I realized I had given away a lot of money. I got angry but thought if I stopped giving people change, no one would talk to me during lunch, so I kept doing it. I got more and more upset so I talked to the school counselor. She helped me realize I continued to give others money so I wouldn't feel lonely. The others were taking advantage of me, but I let them so I wouldn't experience loneliness."

In this example, healthy boundaries would be Rob telling a person who asks for change, "I'll give you money this time, but unless you pay me back I won't do so again in the future." If he continues to set these boundaries with others, they will no longer be able to take advantage of him. As a result he will feel proud of himself for not allowing others to take him for granted. He will be more balanced.

Obese people often feel like others take advantage of them. They do not set healthy personal boundaries for themselves, fearing they will be alone, abandoned, not acknowledged, not included, and not liked. As a result, others do often take advantage of them. If this is to change, Terri, Rob and others like them, must learn to set boundaries.

When an obese person loses weight, they still have emotional needs to be included, to be acknowledged, and to be liked. Their way of getting these needs met sometimes takes on a new look. The newly thin person can still be taken advantage of unless they learn to set healthy boundaries. Losing weight does not have the benefit of automatically instilling healthy behaviors!

Trina said she slept with people whether she was heavy or not because she so badly wanted to feel cared for. She abandoned her personal values to get that need met. She had poor personal boundaries, whether heavy or thin. In therapy, she learned healthier ways to get her needs for acceptance and feeling cared about met without devaluing herself. She learned to set healthy personal boundaries. She spent time with people and engaged in healthy activities. She learned that people wanted to spend time with her because they valued her personality. She didn't need to have sex with people for them to want to be with her.

Gretchen, who went out with her friends while ignoring her husband and children after she lost weight, was an example of a person who switched from having rigid social boundaries before surgery to having few social boundaries after losing weight. "I went from staying home and not having friends when I was fat to feeling taken advantage of by friends after I lost weight and started to go out all the time. I always volunteered to drive; I often bought drinks for everyone and I found myself being the one to make most of the plans for our activities. I realize that after losing weight, even though I felt more attractive, allowed myself to be seen in public, and believed I finally had a lot of friends, I still didn't feel good about myself on the inside. I guess I thought if I didn't pay for drinks when we were out or if I didn't make plans that I would still be left out. I feared my 'friends' didn't actually like me just because I'm me. Doing all of those things was a way to be sure I was included. I ended up letting myself and my family down in the long run. Now I know how to live a balanced social life. I go out with my girlfriends once a week or so. Sometimes I let them buy my lunch. Sometimes I still buy. Sometimes I make plans and they do actually call me when they make plans. I know now that they like me, even if I sometimes decline an invitation. My family is happier because I am home more and I'm happier. I now have respect for myself." Gretchen has learned to set healthy personal boundaries. She has balanced her Social Center.

The healthiest place to be in life, most of the time, is in the middle.

A Balanced Social Life – Skinny or Fat

Whether a person is fat, skinny or somewhere in between, setting healthy personal boundaries is essential for good mental health. It is common for people to swing from one end of the continuum to the other when they are early in recovery from an addiction, when they lose a tremendous amount of weight, or when they alter their life in some other drastic way. Trina and Gretchen are examples of obese people moving from one end of the social continuum before having weight loss surgery to the other end after losing a lot of weight. They had to learn the hard way how to have balance.

That Old Chicken and Egg Thing

So which comes first? Having healthy boundaries or demonstrating balanced behavior? A better question may be, "Does it matter?" The goal is to have both healthy boundaries *and* balanced behavior in all of your Centers of Balance. Sometimes insight can lead to healthy behavior change. But remember: Insight is *not* required for you to change your behavior. Learning about healthy boundaries *can* lead to healthy behaviors and balanced living. However, you can learn about healthy behaviors and implement them, without fully understanding all about personal boundaries. Healthy behavior will result in healthy boundaries.

Bottom line? *Always do the next right thing.* In the case of a post-bariatric patient, this means completing your Gotta Do Ems daily. The GDEs for balancing your Social Center are:

- balance time between your family, friends, and social obligations (this does not necessarily mean giving them all equal time)
- establish healthy boundaries for yourself in relation to others
- maintain personal values in your social interactions
- consider the needs and wants of others involved

Be prepared for personal and social relationships to change after you have weight loss surgery, and especially as you begin to implement new personal boundaries. Your family members and friends are used to you behaving in certain, specific ways. Chances are, as an obese person, you have a long history of living without strong personal boundaries and/ or taking advantage of other people's boundaries. A lack of personal boundaries in your social life results in your being taken advantage of by others. You may volunteer to do (or be convinced to do) things you don't want to do (driving, buying, organizing, etc.) so you will be accepted, invited again, or perceived of as being nice. You may allow yourself to be taken advantage of sexually in order to feel desired, wanted or needed. When you change your behavior and set boundaries (which anyone can do, whether they are fat or thin), others respond, sometimes in ways that will surprise you and sometimes in ways that will anger you or hurt your feelings.

For example, if you are the mom that the PTA president calls every time they need a fund raiser held, what do you think will happen next time they call and you respectfully tell them, "I love helping the school and the PTA, which I do regularly. I'm sorry but I won't be able to do the fundraiser for band uniforms as I have other commitments."? Chances are, the caller will do their best to convince you to do it *just this one time.* Remember, they are accustomed to your obliging them. You'll probably feel like caving in and fulfilling their request. If you do, they are sure to pressure you every time they want you to do something. If you give in, you will feel badly about yourself for not having the strength to stand up for yourself. You may feel guilty at first when you choose to say no when you're asked to do something you don't want to do, but ultimately, you will feel proud of yourself for taking care of your own needs. (That doesn't mean you can't ever help out with projects … that would be demonstrating rigid boundaries. Volunteer to do things when you can and when you want to. Feel free to say "no" to projects when you legitimately don't want to, or don't have time to do them. BALANCE.)

You may lose some friends in the process of learning to set healthy boundaries in your social world. When you start to say "no" to people you believe are your friends and they are not used to it, those who aren't your true friends may fall by the wayside. Let them go, remembering that you are worth having as a friend, even if you don't do things for others on their timetable.

Karen shared her sadness over the loss of someone she thought was a good friend. "My friend Traci and I had done so many things together during the past two years. Our kids were good friends, and they participated in a lot of the same activities. I didn't have many other friends, which is something I always wanted. As I lost weight I started becoming friends with people at the support group. I was happy about meeting new people. I started doing social activities with people besides Traci, even though I considered her to be my best friend and we still did a lot of things together. She started getting mad at me and treating me badly. We finally talked about it. She told me that I didn't have time for her any more and she decided I was not a good friend. She no longer wants to have anything to do with me. I'm really sad about it but realize that I need more than one friend in my life. I hope Traci will eventually come around and be my friend again, but right now, I feel it's best for me to have different people in my life and do social things with others. My husband likes that I have a wider group of friends and so do the kids. We're doing fun things together."

Family members don't always like the changes you make in your social life when you lose weight, feel better physically, and want to get more involved in the world outside your front door. "Tim felt threatened when I started going out with female friends," Doris said. "I was just going for lunch once in a while or to an occasional movie, but he would get mad, saying I didn't have time for him any more. He and I started having a date night once a week, and then he started feeling better about it. I guess he just wanted to be reassured that just because I am now thinner, I won't abandon him."

As you lose weight, you will probably want to be more socially active. Finding ways to include your children, spouse, and other important people in your new activities will make them feel included in your new life. Invite your kids and spouse to go with you to do the social things you did not allow yourself to do when you were heavy. Take a martial arts class or line dancing class together. Go to an art gallery or a museum together. Finding balance in your life means considering the needs of others as well as your own.

No More Go-fers

Your kids and spouses can be especially affected, interpersonally and socially, as you lose weight. When you were at your heaviest weight, you were probably inactive, at least around the house. Your spouse and/ or your kids were probably your very own personal go-fers. "Honey, go-fer this and honey, go-fer that. Bring me a soda. Get me the remote for the TV. Feed the dog. Do the laundry. Go-fer, go-fer, go-fer." You were too tired to get up. It hurt to walk around and do things. After having surgery, you may realize how you took advantage of your family members (like how I snuck that bit about you taking advantage of others in there?) and now you want to take responsibility for your own needs by doing things for yourself. Don't be surprised if your little go-fers feel displaced. Although it is not a healthy role for kids or spouses to be placed in, you may have treated them like they were your personal attendants. Even though they would prefer to get attention from you in healthier ways, they did get attention by fetching you things and doing things for you. When you change your behavior and do things for yourself, your spouse or children lose their role of caregiver to you. You need to be mindful that they still need your attention and appreciation. Make it a point to include them in the things you do around the house, as opposed to doing it yourself all of a sudden. They will enjoy participating with you and being included in your world.

Your social life with your family will change as you lose weight, both inside and outside the home. Make it a positive thing for your entire family. They'll need your help. The changes taking place as a result of your weight loss will be confusing to them.

Confusing to Whom*?*

The changes that take place in your life, internally and socially, will be confusing to you, as well. At times you will be scared about people's reactions to your weight loss. Stella marveled, "People who previously would not give me the time of day were all of sudden acting like we were best friends. At first I liked it. It reminded me of when I was in high school and wanted the 'popular people' to like me. Now sometimes I get mad when people who used to ignore me suddenly want to chat with me. I want to know why I wasn't good enough for them when I was heavy. I feel angry just thinking about it. Overall, though, it feels good to have people be more receptive to me. I'm sure it's due in part to the fact that I'm thinner now, but it may also have to do with the fact that I am more approachable than I was before I lost the weight. *I* probably talk to people now that I didn't talk to before, as well."

The feelings you experience as people respond to you differently can be intoxicating. "I'll never forget what it was like when a guy at work who I had a crush on first noticed me," Jackie said. "I saw him start to look at me when I was walking down the hall. One day he said hello as we passed. Pretty soon he was stopping by my desk to talk. I thought I was going to die from happiness every time he spoke to me."

Preston said, "The coolest thing for me was when I started getting chosen for teams at tennis league. I was used to being the one who wasn't picked until the very end. Now, I get picked early on when the captains choose teams. It inspires me to work even harder at my tennis game, as well as improving my health and building my social circle."

Mad, sad, glad and scared. You'll feel them all in relation to your weight loss and the changes in your social life.

To Tell or Not to Tell

A number of years ago, I was watching my seven-year-old nephew standing alone in a lake, minding his own business. Apparently thinking out loud, he shouted, "To be or not to be… THAT IS A QUESTION." Not "that is *the* question," as Shakespeare wrote, but *a* question. "To tell or not to tell" (about your surgery) is also *a* question.

There are a number of things to consider in determining whether or not to tell people about your bariatric surgery:

- Who do you tell?
- When do you tell them?
- Who needs to know?
- Who has a right to know?
- Who do you *want* to tell?
- Who do you *not* want to tell?

Obviously, your spouse/partner, children, parents, siblings, friends, bosses, and coworkers are likely to be aware of your weight loss after surgery, but you need to take some very important things into consideration before talking about your decision to have bariatric surgery:

Who really needs to know? Some people need to know about your weight loss surgery, simply for general health reasons. If there are complications or some sort of medical emergency related (or unrelated) to your surgery, someone close to you will have to tell the medical professionals involved in your care that you had bariatric surgery. Obviously, the fact that you had bariatric surgery will be in your medical records, but having someone close to you aware of your medical situation is a good idea.

Who will genuinely support you? One thing is certain, it is essential to have the emotional support of people you trust following bariatric surgery, whether that is a friend, family member, or spouse. You will need physical *and* emotional support from this person as time goes by. There will be times when you are sad or angry or upset as you grieve not being able to eat like you want to. You will be tempted to eat foods that are disagreeable to post-bariatric patients. The trusted people in your support system can help you through these times by encouraging you to eat the right things, by distracting you when you have "head hunger," by cheering you on through the rough spots, and by celebrating with you in your many successes. For these reasons and more, the person most actively involved in your life on a day-to-day basis is someone you need to tell about your surgery.

On the other hand, just because people are involved in your life does not mean they necessarily need to know about your surgery. Before you consider telling each person, you need to decide just how supportive they will be if they know. Sadly, sometimes family members or even spouses may sabotage your success following surgery. You may need to refrain from telling some people who are close to you. For example, if a sibling, other relative or friend engages in some sort of rivalry with you, whether spoken or unspoken, it may be wise not to tell them you are having weight loss surgery, especially if they are the type who "always needs to win." Consciously or unconsciously, they might try to sabotage your success.

"My older sister, who has always had a weight problem, would tempt me to eat if she knew about my surgery," Stella said. "She would ask me to go to dinner at my old favorite buffet restaurant. She would bring me fattening desserts or eat luscious but dangerous foods in front of me. She would talk about food in my presence. When a good friend of hers had bypass surgery, my sister claimed to be supportive of her, but I saw her do all of those sabotaging behaviors."

Do your children need to know? It depends on their age and their ability to understand obesity and about the surgery. If you choose to tell your children, let them be part of the entire process. Educate them about obesity, its causes and consequences. Have them attend the information sessions about the surgery and about postsurgical living. Let them meet your surgeon and ask questions. Your children may be frightened about the surgery. They may have heard "horror stories" on television about bariatric surgery. It is essential for them to have factual information. If you choose to tell your children, make the recovery from obesity a family affair. Cook healthy meals with your children. Become active with them by walking, riding bicycles, going to the gym, and playing ball together. You will be helping yourself and helping them develop healthy behaviors.

What about telling your boss and co-workers? Again, it depends. How long will you be away from work? If your weight-loss procedure requires you to be away from your job for many weeks, you may have to inform someone from the office about the reason for your absence. If you work in an environment where gossip at the water cooler is the reason people go to work in the first place, be extremely selective about who you tell. Be prepared, though. The minute you tell one or two people, it won't be long before everyone in your office – and probably the two or three offices down the hall – knows "the big news." If you choose not to tell co-workers, and they start asking questions as you lose weight, simply share with them that you have changed your eating and exercise behaviors. That *is* the truth! It is quite possible to return to work, go out to lunch with your co-workers, and survive the donut-filled break room without anyone on the job site knowing you had bariatric surgery.

The bottom line is that you only want to tell people who will support you throughout the process. An important issue surrounding whether you choose "To Tell or Not to Tell" is related to those good old boundaries we discussed earlier in the chapter. It is never a good idea to tell someone your whole life story – to include the issue of bariatric surgery – until you know them and can trust them. I always suggest to people that if someone tells you their entire life story within the first ten minutes of meeting you… run like crazy – in the opposite direction! Having healthy emotional boundaries means you disclose personal information sparingly to persons who have earned your trust. (Being a family member does not automatically guarantee trustworthiness.)

Your decision to have bariatric surgery is a personal one. Your decision to share the information is equally personal. Be smart. Choose to tell those persons you can count on to genuinely support you in the rough times and to celebrate with you as you achieve your personal goals! Saboteurs, unfortunately, come in the form of intimates and strangers.

Stella chose not to tell her sister about her decision to have weight-loss surgery based on observing her sister's sabotaging behavior toward a friend who had a similar procedure. Karen's friendship with Traci ended as Karen's social interactions changed following her weight loss. Time after time clients tell me stories about their relationships with family members and friends changing as they lose weight. Many times my clients are surprised and hurt, noting, "I thought they were happy for me." Marriages, too, are very often challenged when one partner experiences a drastic change like significant weight loss.

Just as you will have emotional reactions to your weight loss, so will family members and friends. Even though they may genuinely be happy for you, they also have emotional reactions they don't anticipate, such as:

- jealousy about the way people look at you after you have lost weight
- envy that they are not getting the same amount of attention as you
- anger because you participate in more social activities as a thin person and are leaving home more often
- fear (on the part of spouses or significant others) that you will become romantically interested in someone else
- irritation as you learn to set healthy boundaries and start saying "no"
- annoyance at your seeming obsession with weight loss issues
- negativity and spite from family members and others for all of the above reasons

"You've Changed"

No words could be more accurate when said in relation to a person who has lost more than 100 pounds in a year! The physical changes are only part of the picture, as anyone who has been in that position knows. As this book emphasizes, every area of a person's life changes after they have weight loss surgery. When friends, family members, children, and spouses say "You've changed" they also mean that your relationship with them has changed.

Mary Ann complained, "My husband and I argue all the time since I lost weight. He's mad if I wear something he thinks is too "sexy," so we fight about that. He argues if I want to go anywhere, even if I ask him to come with me, and we get into it about that. We argue about my decision to go to the gym on the way home from work. We're constantly bickering!" As Mary Ann's body changed, so did her relationship with her husband. I reminded her that the changes in her body were positive because her health was greatly improved, as was her self-image. We discussed the fact that her husband was likely experiencing feelings of insecurity, jealousy, and fear. I encouraged Mary Ann to talk with him about the fact that it is normal for him to have these feelings. Rather than argue about it, they could choose to identify their feelings and the needs associated with them. Her husband would need reassurance that Mary Ann loved him and would continue to love him no matter how much weight she lost. He needed affirmation that she still wanted to spend time with him.

The people you love go through changes in response to the changes you make following weight loss. They too, experience new thoughts, feelings and behaviors in relation to your weight loss. Consider their feelings and their needs in this process. It is easy to become (or remain) overly self-focused as you lose weight and experience the world in different ways.

I also told Mary Ann something that I learned from a therapist a long time ago: "If you stop arguing with him there won't be an argument." In other words, if her husband is argumentative, Mary Ann could choose to respond calmly and refuse to argue back, in which case, there would be no argument! Effective communication skills and good listening skills are essential to balancing the Social Center.

Communicating: The Hardest Easy Thing to Do

In our social relationships we communicate all the time. Verbally and nonverbally. We learn to talk in the first years of our life. It's easy to talk! Why then, is it so difficult to communicate effectively even when we are well into our adult lives? Ineffective communication causes imbalance in our Social Centers because people misunderstand one another, fail to make their needs and wants known, and focus too much on another person's behavior. People retreat from one another when these things happen. Marriages fail and friendships end because of ineffective communication.

As long as so many things are changing for the positive in your world while you lose weight, you might as well improve your communication skills in the process. Doing so will help you deal effectively with your changing social relationships following weight loss.

Effective listening means paying attention to more than the words a person uses. Anna Beth gave a good example of the importance of listening to both the words she used and the feelings she was experiencing when she talked with her husband. "I had lost 75 pounds and was feeling good about myself, but I hadn't seen many people from my husband's office since my surgery. We were expected to attend their holiday party. I continued to make comments to my husband about not being excited about the party and wishing we had a good excuse to get out of going. After hearing me talk like this for several days, my husband sat me down, took my hands, and said, 'Honey, it sounds like you are anxious and fearful about going to this party. Are you afraid they'll ask questions, or are you nervous about getting a lot of attention in public?' I couldn't believe it! He pointed out the feelings I hadn't even acknowledged I was experiencing! That helped me talk about those feelings with him. I was still nervous about going to the party, but it helped being able to talk about it."

If Anna Beth's husband had just listened to her words, he may have asked questions like, "Why don't you want to go? You know all of these people. What's the big deal?" Questions like this could easily have led to an argument. Fortunately, her husband listened to her words *and* her unspoken, underlying feelings. He was able to hear her anxiety and fear, even though she hadn't used those words. Anna Beth felt understood by him, which led to a good discussion about her fear and anxiety.

When we speak to others we want them to hear both what we say *and* how we feel. When others speak to us, they want the same. When we let them know that we hear what they are saying *and* how they feel, they feel deeply understood. We all want that.

Practice listening to the words and feelings people convey to you. When your child says, "I hate my teacher!" say to your child, "Wow! You hate your teacher. You sound really angry!" This sort of response encourages the child to tell you more. If you said something like, "It's not nice to hate someone," your child is being told her feelings are bad or wrong. Your child wants to tell you the reasons she "hates" her teacher. Doing so will be a lot easier if you focus on how your child is feeling.

Practice listening for the feeling behind people's words. When others talk to you, say to yourself, "Based on what this person is saying and how they are saying it, how is this person feeling?" Try responding to both the words they use and how you think they feel. Doing so will help others open up more and discuss the issue. When you talk to others, ask yourself "What am I feeling?" and add that to your comment. For example, say "We're having dinner with my husband's entire family next week. I haven't lost any weight since we saw them last. I'm scared they will judge me." This will help the person you're talking to address what's really important, which is your fear of being judged. If you simply say, "We're having dinner with my husband's entire family next week. I really dread it," your friend may miss what you are trying to say. She may go off on a completely different direction in her response to you: "Yeah, I'll bet. The way you described his sister, I would be dreading it too." You might find yourself frustrated with your friend, thinking she doesn't understand. Help people out when you talk to them. Give them words and your feelings. Teach your friends and family to communicate this way. You'll be amazed at how much more productive conversations become, how much less arguing you do, and how much more you feel genuinely understood by others.

"I" Messages

Chances are good you've read at least one article on "I" messages or have heard about them on a talk show. "I" messages are a great communication tool, and yet it's fascinating to see how people misuse them! The idea behind using "I" messages is to keep the focus on how "I" think, how "I" feel, and what "I" observe. Read these two examples of Sally talking to her husband:

Example 1: "Honey, there's something I want to talk with you about. Since you lost 150 pounds, I have noticed a lot of changes, many of them positive, which we have talked about in the past two years. However, in the past few months you have been flirting like crazy with other women. I think you are making a fool of yourself and should be ashamed."

Example 2: "Honey, there's something I want to talk with you about. Since you lost 150 pounds, I have noticed a lot of changes, many of them positive, which we have talked about in the past two years. However, in the past few months it seems to me like you have been flirting with other women. I wonder if I am being overly sensitive or if you may not be aware that you're flirting. When I see you do that, I feel insecure. I don't want to make a big deal out of this but I wanted you to know what I have observed and how I feel. Can we talk more about this?"

If you were Sally's husband, how would you feel if you heard your wife use the words in Example #1? Defensive, embarrassed, accused, angry, and hurt? "I" messages are supposed to be about the *speaker's* thoughts, feelings and observations. They are not supposed to be a way to shame someone else. In Example #2, Sally's husband is less likely to feel attacked. Sally took responsibility for sharing her thoughts, feelings, and observations in an appropriate way.

Here are some other examples of positive and negative uses of "I" messages. Pay attention to how you would feel if you received these messages:

Positive: "When you bring junk food into the house after you have agreed not to, I feel betrayed."

Negative: "You brought junk food home. You obviously don't care if I am successful at losing weight. I feel like you lied to me about not bringing junk food in the house." (NOTE: A feeling word should follow "I feel"... sad, mad, glad, etc.)

Positive: "I feel embarrassed when you make jokes about my surgery when we are out with our friends. I would appreciate if you would stop doing that."

Negative: "You embarrass me when we're with our friends. I think you're a jerk. You need to stop." (Note that "I think," was followed by "you" and a criticism; a misuse of "I" messages).

Positive: "When you ask me to drive to the majority of our outings, I feel taken advantage of. I would appreciate if we took turns driving or shared the cost of gas."

Negative: "I'm sick of you taking advantage of me. You drive for a change."

The point is to use "I" messages to focus on your own thoughts, your own feelings, and your own observations. Even if the person you're talking to doesn't respond well to what you say, you are making an effort to communicate in a positive way.

Fair Fighting

If you do get into a disagreement with someone in your social circles, what makes for a fair fight? The basics for fair fighting include:

- Talk about one issue at a time, the one at hand. Don't bring up past arguments.
- Directly state what your concern is, using "I" language and include how you feel.

- Avoid blaming, name-calling, personal attacks, sarcasm, and threats.
- Take a timeout if you are getting too worked up; tell the person you need to take a break and resume the discussion in an agreed-upon amount of time.
- Avoid the words "Why," "Never," and "Always"
- Have your discussion in private; keeps kids and others out of it.
- Allow both parties equal time.
- Take responsibility for your part in the situation.
- Accept apologies.

When emotions are intense, it can be difficult to fight fairly. Make the effort. The best way to keep fighting calm is to try to see the situation from the other person's perspective. Let's use the example of Sally who feels insecure, worrying that her husband is flirting with other women. Let's say her husband said to her, "Sally. I have no idea what you're talking about! If I have been flirting with other women I'm not aware of it. I know I spoke to women at the office party last week, but it didn't feel flirtatious to me."

The discussion would probably go smoothly if Sally said something like, "Obviously, this has surprised you. You seem to be aware that you were talking to other women. Since you look so great after losing weight, it would make sense to me that getting attention from other women would feel good. I know that I have been feeling vulnerable. Maybe you weren't flirting, and I mistook what I saw because I am feeling insecure. I know you love me and wouldn't want to hurt me intentionally. I wanted to bring this up so we could talk about it. I guess I need reassurance."

Sally's husband could help by acknowledging where she was coming from by saying, "Honey, I want you to know that I understand how you could mistake what you saw as flirting. It's nice that you recognize that it feels good to have attention after losing weight. But I don't want or need flirtation from other women. I love you and enjoy when we flirt together. I will be careful when I talk to women to make sure I am not being flirtatious. I don't want to come across that way. Thank you for bringing it to my attention."

Sadly, that's not the way most of us learned to argue. We rarely hear one another as we're focused on defending our own position when we argue. Do yourself a favor and work at letting the other person know you are attempting to understand their position. It can make a tremendous difference in resolving disagreements with less heartache and in less time.

Mind Reading

We want other people to be able to read our minds. They can't. It will never happen. You can't read theirs either. So "get over it" if you're one of those people who say anything even close to "Why do I have to tell him/her? He/she should just know!" People think in very different ways. You might think that your husband should just know what to do to help you by looking around the room at the "obvious" disaster you see. When he asks you, "What can I do to help?" just tell him specifically what you want him to do instead of firing away, "What do you mean what can you do to help?! Can't you see this place is a disaster?! Just pick something and start cleaning up!" Instead, try, "Well, the toys need to be picked up and the dishes need to be done. Which would you rather do?"

You must also take responsibility for making your thoughts known. For example, your teenagers may not understand the importance of keeping junk food out of the house after you have weight loss surgery. You think they should know that without having to be told. Tell them, gently but firmly, "I understand that you can have junk food now and then and it won't harm you. But having that sort of food around the house is dangerous for me. Please eat your junk food when you're out with your friends so we don't have it in the house. I would really appreciate your help."

If former friends have begun to distance themselves from you and it upsets you, make your feelings and needs known. "Maggie, lately it seems like we've been drifting apart. I don't know if I'm overreacting but I'm sad because your friendship means a lot to me. I want to talk about anything that may be coming between us that results in our not spending time together."

It takes courage and determination to say things you are thinking and feeling. It is hard to lay your thoughts and feelings on the table. It can be even more difficult to ask for help.

Learning to Ask for Help

A lot of people find it difficult to ask for help. Obese people are notorious for doing things for others. As we've seen, doing things for others has a personal benefit of meeting one's need for acceptance or being included. Regardless, it is much easier for obese people to do things for others than it is for them to ask for help (except, maybe, at home, where spouses and children may be personal go-fers).

Asking for help can mean a lot of things. "Could you please give me a lift home after the support group meeting?" "I'm not sure how to get through times when I have a strong craving for something chocolaty and gooey. How do *you* do that?" "Would you like to get a group together and order a shipment of protein shakes? They're less expensive if we buy them in large quantities."

What makes it difficult to ask for help? Underneath the reasons for not asking for help lie psychological insecurities. "I don't want to bother anyone" may really mean, "I don't think I'm important enough to bother with." "I was taught to do things for myself" might really mean, "I'm too proud to ask for help."

Ironically, when asked to help someone else, are you the first person to volunteer? What makes it okay, in your book, for someone else to ask for help while it's not okay for you to do the same? Is that pride? Arrogance? Insecurity? Learning to ask for help is essential for balancing your Social Center. Balance requires that you learn to give and to receive. Just like you enjoy helping others, they, too, like to be of service to you. Let them!

Unhealthy Communication = Imbalance and Bad Habits

The weeks and months following weight loss surgery are a time of change for you, the patient, and for everyone closely associated with you. Your Social Center is greatly affected after you have weight loss surgery. If your Social Center gets stuck off balance, you may return to old eating habits out of frustration.

Jim explained, "My wife and I seemed to grow further and further apart after I began losing weight. We would bicker a lot. We seemed unable to talk for any length of time without arguing. After months of struggling, I noticed I would often go to the convenience store after we would argue. I gained 10 pounds before I identified the pattern. Fortunately, she agreed to go to couple's therapy. We're now learning how to talk and get through tough issues. I am learning healthier ways of dealing with frustration rather than turning to food again."

Samantha's Social Center was most imbalanced at the office. "I used to go to lunch with the gang every day. After having surgery, I made the decision to bring my lunch to work and eat it in the break room every day. I started feeling like I wasn't a part of the group anymore. Instead of talking to my friends at the office and letting them know I was feeling insecure, I started to go to the restaurants again for lunch. It wasn't long before my weight started to increase. I knew I couldn't continue to go out for lunch every day and I was scared of losing my friends. I finally got up the courage to talk to my closest friends. Now some of them bring their lunch to the office a couple of days a week. That helps a lot. Telling them how I felt was good for me too. It's getting much easier for me to ask for help from my family members and to be more direct with my husband. I'm excited about my new communication abilities!"

Regress Toward the Mean

I hated taking Statistics classes! My mind doesn't naturally think that way and so it was always difficult for me to understand much in those classes. One of the things that sticks in my mind is "regress toward the mean," which has something to do with averages. It means finding Balance, staying away from the extremes.

A balanced Social Center requires being able to set healthy boundaries with other people. This is a skill that needs to be learned, along with practicing healthy communication. Sustaining your weight loss depends on your being able to set healthy social boundaries. If you are unable to do so, negative thoughts, negative feelings and unhealthy behaviors lead to self sabotage and often to weight regain as food is again used as a balm to soothe these old patterns.

A balanced Social Center as part of a healthy lifestyle is essential for establishing and maintaining a balanced Enterprise Center. Your life legacy is encompassed in this self-actualizing Center.

Chapter 6: End of Chapter Exercises

Balance Brainwork

1. Make a list of your current social activities. For each activity, note your reason(s) for participating in it. (Is it something you participate in because you want to or because you feel you "should?")
2. If your life is too busy, decide on two activities you will drop.
3. If your life has too few social activities, make a list of five things you are interested in being a part of.
4. Write about how you feel in social situations. Are you preoccupied with how you look? Do you think others are looking at you? Do you fear others are judging you? Are you looking at/judging others? Do you enjoy social situations? Which ones do you like most/least? How does your weight influence the way you feel in social situations?
5. In what ways have you been negatively self-involved when it comes to your social life? Have you ignored family to be socially involved as a way to overcompensate for obesity? Have you neglected friends and family in social ways by hiding at home because of obesity?

Balance Busters

For each of the negative thought statements that follow, write down the positive statement to replace it.

Example:
Negative statement: "I hate feeling like people are judging me when I'm in a social setting." Positive statement: "I will choose to think people are seeing and thinking about my best qualities when I am in public."

Negative statement: "My family is embarrassed by me when we go to public places together." Positive statement: _____

_____.

Negative statement: "I would rather stay home alone than expose myself to ridicule in public." Positive statement: _____

_____.

Balance Boosters

When you are asked to be on a committee, participate in a parenting activity, or be part of a charity organization, think about how you will respond. For example, "Let me give this some thought, look over my calendar and get back to you." Take time to decide if you actually want to participate in the activity rather than responding "yes" out of habit. Before deciding, ask yourself the following questions: "Is this an activity I would enjoy?" "Is this an activity important to me or someone in my family?" "Do I have time to do this?" "Will I have time to take care of my health and my priorities if I add this activity to my life?"

If you have avoided social activities because of your weight, make a chart with the following information for activities you would enjoy taking part in:
- group/social activity
- date/time of meeting or activity
- contact information to learn more about the activity
- date by which you will obtain information on this activity
- date by which you will participate in this activity.

The Best of the Best

- "Don't walk in front of me, I may not follow. Don't walk behind me, I may not lead. Just walk beside me and be my friend." - Albert Camus
- "The only way to have a friend is to be one." - Ralph Waldo Emerson
- "A friend is one who knows us, but loves us anyway." - Fr. Jerome Cummings
- "Remember, the greatest gift is not found in a store nor under a tree, but in the hearts of true friends."- Cindy Lew
- "Hold a true friend with both your hands." - Nigerian Proverb
- "A faithful friend is the medicine of life." - Apocrypha

- "Friendship multiplies the good of life and divides the evil."
  - Baltasar Gracian (1647)

Cardinal Convictions

Write three Cardinal Convictions you will make part of your daily self-talk designed to remind yourself that participating in healthy social activities is essential to your long term goal of sustained weight loss. For example: "I will participate in social activities that I enjoy, that are beneficial to me and that fit into my schedule."

Chapter 7

When I Grow Up: Your Enterprise Center

"Happiness comes from spiritual wealth, not material wealth. Happiness comes from giving, not getting. If we try hard to bring happiness to others, we cannot stop it from coming to us also. To get joy, we must give it, and to keep joy, we must scatter it."

-- John Templeton

Ask a child what she or he wants to be as an adult, and you will probably hear responses such as:

- I want to be a teacher.
- I want to be a fire fighter.
- I want to be a professional baseball player.
- I want to be a rock star.
- I want to be a mommy/daddy.

How would you have responded to that question? What did you want "to be" when you grew up? For most of us, childhood dreams are replaced by reality. Many of us dreamed of careers involving fame and fortune; few people have the talent (or money or connections) to actually be professional athletes, singers, or movie stars. I wanted to be Cinderella, the Cinderella from the Rogers & Hammerstein musical that aired on television once a year. It was a big deal in our house when those once-a-year special productions came on TV. The *Wizard of Oz* was the biggie to most people, but for me, the night *Cinderella* aired was the best night of the year. I wanted to be her. I physically ached to be her. I could sing all of the songs—in fact I can still sing those songs word for word. I can also still feel the yearning in my heart as that 10-year-old

147

girl to be transformed into the astonishingly beautiful Cinderella on the night of the ball.

I wanted Price Charming to watch me, bedazzled, as I made my way down a wide staircase, dressed in the most gorgeous gown ever to be worn, adorned in sparkling jewels, smiling coyly as I ever-so-slowly stepped toward him. I wanted my Prince to gaze adoringly into my eyes, unable to take his eyes off me for even a second, amazed at my beauty. I wanted him to seek me out and carry me away to my happily-ever-after. Did I get that? (Actually, my husband is quite a prince, but that's another book.) I sure as heck don't get to wear dazzling gowns every day, and my prince doesn't gaze lovingly into my eyes every second of the day!

I also wanted to be a writer. My mother recently gave me a box of "treasures" she kept from my childhood. In it was a letter I wrote to some unknown person. The letter said, "I would like to be an author. I can't draw very well but I like to write. Please let me know how to print a book."

Think back to yourself as a young person. What did you want to be when you grew up? What sort of personal life did you want to have? Many of us wanted to be married and have children, to have our own home, to do good things in our communities, to have enjoyable hobbies, and to have a stable job that provided for our family, a job we enjoyed going to every day.

Our jobs, our hobbies, our community involvement, and the ways we choose to develop our minds make up our Enterprise Center. A balanced Enterprise Center leads to the fulfillment and joy of leaving a positive and meaningful legacy.

Just as it does with all the other centers, obesity causes imbalance in the Enterprise Center. Certainly, few people daydream of themselves being obese when they grow up. Being obese interferes with your hopes and dreams. It prevents you from living up to your abilities and may restrict you from working in a career field you would love. Obesity may prevent you from conceiving a child. Obesity makes it difficult, if not impossible, for you to follow dreams of travel.

The preceding chapters have left no doubt of the negative impact obesity has on a person's life. Obesity decreases self-esteem. It generates negative thoughts, feelings, and behaviors. Being obese interferes with intimate and casual relationships and decreases our ability and willingness to be socially involved. Being obese prevents people from having the ultimate relationships with God, with self, and with others, and it causes imbalance in your efforts to realize your dreams and aspirations.

How has your obesity caused imbalance in your Enterprise Center? To determine this, answer the following questions:

- Am I working in my career field of choice?
- Do I make as much money as I am capable of making?
- Do I actively participate in community/volunteer work?
- Am I regularly improving my mind through continuing education, reading, watching educational television, etc.?
- Am I involved in the lives of my children or loved ones, attending their concerts, sporting events, etc.?
- Do I support my community by my active involvement in activities and events?
- Do I participate in healthy hobbies of my own interest?

For the questions you answered "No" to, ask yourself, "How has my obesity interfered in this?" Be honest with yourself. Ask people you trust to give you their opinions about how your obesity has interfered with being involved in the above activities.

Michael, a telephone marketer, told me, "I hated facing the fact that my obesity affected every area of my life. It hurt to admit that all of my Centers were off balance. I hate my job as a telephone marketer. I always wanted to be a photographer for sporting events. I even got a degree in photographic journalism. But I got too fat to run up and down ball fields taking action shots. I rarely go to my niece and nephews' sporting events, either, although I love those kids – and the sports! I'm embarrassed about being so large and I fear people are talking badly about me, so I stay away from crowds. I don't want to embarrass the kids by being 'the fat uncle', either. I used to be active in sports myself. Being fat has prevented me from continuing those things. My goal is to start a summer program for obese teens and help them lose weight in fun, active ways so they don't have to miss out on so much, like I have."

Your Career

Being asked "What do you do?" has always irritated me. I get frustrated because if often seems that to know my line of work (or my husband's) is a way of determining my worth. I have very mixed feelings about our work being associated with who we are. In many cases, what we do is truly a part of who we are. For example, my work as a psychologist incorporates much of who I am. I am inquisitive, compassionate, and people-oriented, in my work and in general. But if I hadn't had the opportunity to go to school and get the education I needed to be a psychologist, I would still be innately inquisitive, compassionate, and people-oriented. I don't want my work title to be the measure by which a person "judges" me.

Whether or not the essence of who you are is expressed through your work, it is important to find value in who you are more than in what you do. In other words, self worth does not depend on a particular title, just as how you feel about yourself does not have to be defined by the number on the scale. Regardless of your job title, or how much you weigh, you are you! You have a unique blend of personality traits, talents, abilities, ideas, sense of humor, and your very own experiences in life that makes you different from every other person who has ever lived. How you choose to use this combination of traits and experiences is up to you.

Choice! What Choice?

"I *had* to be a physician because my parents expected me to be one."

"Our family business is plumbing. I had no choice but to follow in my dad's and granddad's footsteps."

"I wanted to dance in a dance troupe, but I was too heavy to be a professional dancer."

"Every female in my family is a nurse. I just figured that's what I was supposed to do."

"Being fat made me want to hide, so I work in a warehouse in a cubicle."

Did you choose your career or did someone else choose it for you? Has being obese prevented you from following your career dreams? Working in a career you don't like that was chosen for you by someone else results in personal unhappiness, resentment and imbalance in your Centers. Choosing work that you do not like because you are obese also results in an unhappy, angry, imbalanced existence.

Individuation

Individuation is the process of emotionally emancipating yourself from your parents--in other words, being able to say "No" to your parents without feeling guilty. I'll bet you think you have already individuated. I hope you have, although many people in their 40s, 50s and 60s have never accomplished this important developmental task. Try answering these questions:

- Are you in a job because your parents encouraged (or pressured) you to pursue it?
- Do you struggle at holidays, making sure you see everyone so no one has hurt feelings - even though you are miserable trying to get everywhere?
- Are you able to tell your parents "No" without feeling guilty? *Without feeling guilty?*

Individuating means being able to set healthy boundaries with parents and other family members. This is a difficult process because so many emotions are involved. Everyone, whether they are willing to admit it or not, wants acknowledgement, affirmation, and approval from their parents. People sometimes go to ridiculous lengths at their own expense to please their parents; these people are usually angry, resentful, and unbalanced.

Obese people often fail to set healthy boundaries with others in order to be included, liked, or approved of. Learning to set healthy boundaries is a process we develop over time. As you lose weight, you will need a jump-start course in setting boundaries in order to remain true to your goals of losing weight and becoming balanced.

Parents, Obesity and Careers

If you do not already love what you are doing for work, answer these questions:

- What would I love to do for a career?
- Where would my talents be best utilized?
- What type of career would I find enjoyable?
- What kind of work would provide me with personal fulfillment?
- What prevents me from doing the kind of work I would love, that would utilize my talents, interests, and abilities and provide me with a sense of personal fulfillment?

You may discover, as you think about these questions, that your parents or other significant people in your life have given you messages about what you were or were not capable of doing. "I was told that I was 'not college material,'" Linda said. "It never occurred to me to apply to college because that's the message I was given all my life." Rick said, "I was told that fat people would not be accepted as news anchors, so I didn't follow my dreams." You can combat these kinds of messages using the techniques described in the preceding chapters. Messages like this can be difficult to overcome and may require working with a professional. What's most important is that you talk about your feelings related to the path you have followed. You can talk with a friend, your partner, your parents, or a therapist. It's imperative to do the work of letting go of negative thoughts and feelings about your abilities that you have carried around for such a long time!

Reality Check

Perhaps you are thinking: "Get real. I have three kids in school and a pile of student loans myself. I have a job, and I'm stuck in it. The bills have to be paid, and I can't be selfish and just quit what I'm doing and do what I 'like' because it will make me 'happy.'"

Of course you need to be responsible and take care of your children and financial obligations. But you can still take the time to consider what kind of work you would be happiest and most fulfilled doing. This process may bring up psychological issues such as a fear of failure, fear of success, or worries about what other people might think. As you determine what your dream job would be, you may begin to recognize what stands in your way of pursuing that dream, and to determine if you can or want to work toward overcoming any obstacles, including your weight, that prevent you from fulfilling that dream.

Hobbies and Community Involvement

You may be able to realize your dream job through hobbies or community service if you decide it does not make sense for you to pursue a formal career in the field.

"I always wanted to be a financial consultant," Valerie said. "My weight was one thing that prevented me from pursuing work in that field. I figured people wouldn't take anything I had to say seriously because I am obese. I figured they would think I couldn't take control of my own life so I wouldn't be able to advise them in theirs. After having surgery, I promised myself to pursue personal goals. I do think people will respect me more and take me more seriously now that I am losing weight. I guess the truth is, I respect myself more for taking charge of my health. I have started offering free financial advising to the people at my church. It will give me a way to share my talents and to realize my goals, and the experience will be tremendous."

"I always wanted to be an actor in community theatre," Victor said. "But being fat made getting up on stage too frightening a prospect for me. At 350 pounds, I didn't have the courage or confidence to get up in front of an audience. Now that I weigh 190 pounds, I have decided to try out for the local performing group. Losing weight has given me the courage to follow my dream of acting."

I Wanna ...

What hobbies or adventures do you dream about participating in during your lifetime? What things have you told your best friend you really want to do "some day?" Do you want to want to sky-dive, parasail, go on a safari, tour every National Park in the country, ride on the Nile, take an Alaskan cruise, tour history museums, search for Civil War relics on battlefields, run a 10K, home school your grandchildren, volunteer on a medical mission to Haiti, start a homeless shelter, or snorkel in the Bahamas?

Balance your Enterprise Center by making a list of the things you "wanna do," set goals toward doing them, and enjoy! Don't live for "someday," because someday won't come unless you make it happen!

You Can't Keep It If You Don't Give It Away

Alcoholics Anonymous has hundreds of truisms such as "You can't keep it if you don't give it away." In AA, this means in order for you to remain sober, you must share with others what you have learned in AA about how to live a sober life. Newcomers depend on old-timers to teach them how to live a healthy life free from alcohol. The old-timers benefit as much as the newcomers when they share how they have overcome their alcoholism. Sharing our talents and gifts with others is a "Win-Win" proposition, to be sure.

As a postsurgical bariatric patient who is successfully losing weight, you will benefit by sharing your knowledge with others who are preparing for surgery and with those who have recently had surgery. You understand what they are experiencing, both cognitively and emotionally. You can encourage them through the difficult times and celebrate with them as they meet milestones in their recovery from obesity. Talk with the newcomers at your local support group meetings. Share your wisdom on websites and in chat rooms for bariatric patients. As you encourage, educate, and inspire others, you validate your own victories and keep your own flame of endurance burning! Balance in your life and helping others find balance in theirs is definitely a win-win situation.

Try to volunteer in your community as you make changes in your life coinciding with your weight loss. Use your talents, your wisdom, your creativity, your experiences, and your YOU-ness to contribute to the lives of others. This is how to balance your Enterprise Center and leave a positive legacy.

The Pursuit of Happiness

The Declaration of Independence says that people "are endowed by their Creator with certain inalienable rights, that among these are Life, Liberty and the pursuit of Happiness." Notice that the verbiage does not suggest a *guarantee of happiness*. We have a right to the *pursuit* of happiness. No one *owes* us happiness. We have the right to the *pursuit* of happiness.

What are you doing to pursue your own happiness? What stands in your way of being happy?

What is Happy?

"Happy" is what obese people tell me they expect to feel when they have lost weight. Admit it ... you've said it yourself. "When I'm thin, I'll be happy." In other words, thin equals happy. How happy do some of the super-thin celebrities seem to you? The myth that being thin equals being happy is simply wishful thinking. You have probably already experienced the letdown of having lost a significant amount of weight at some point in the past and were disillusioned because you were not instantly happy. An expectant mother looks forward to meeting her baby and being a mother, expecting nothing but joy when that baby bundle finally arrives. In reality, she may experience significant depression after the birth of her child. When you actually get thin, or when a new mother gives birth, there is sometimes an emotional letdown. The dream of living as a confident thin person, a perfectly content new parent, or a blissfully happy newlywed is replaced by the reality that life is just life. Fantasy is not reality. *Thin does not equal happy.* Thin *you* equals fat *you* minus excess weight: the same you with the same thoughts about self, the same childhood history, the same memories, the same insecurities, the same doubts, the same fears, the same strengths. The same you without excess pounds.

"Happiness" is a feeling, a temporary state of being, a mood, a state of mind. Happy suggests euphoria or a heightened state of joy. Happiness is a feeling we experience in bursts. It is not realistic to expect to feel happy all day every day. Contentment is a more realistic goal. Contentment is being at peace with the way things are.

Mostly Well

Americans, it seems to me, are unappreciative of the abundance we have in our lives. We bemoan such little things: our second car is in the shop, our TV/VCR/DVD is in need of repair, our central air conditioning is temporarily not working, our boss is on our case, the big roller coaster at the amusement park is closed for repair, the traffic is annoying, there was no Christmas bonus last year, the latest video game system is out of stock, our cell phone is on the fritz, the fax machine is jammed, and on and on and on.

A wise professor I once had used to say, "Enjoy your pain!" He meant to be grateful for whatever problems we have because most of our "problems" aren't so bad. As the story goes, if everyone in the neighborhood brought his or her problems to the village green, hung all of their problems on a clothes line, and then chose which problems to take home, most people would choose to take home the same problems they brought with them.

In this country, we don't really know what problems are in comparison to people in countries where women see husbands killed in front of them, husbands see wives and daughters raped in front of them, children are taken from parents and sold as sex slaves, babies have no access to vaccinations, parents have no food or means of obtaining food for their families, living quarters are infested by insects and rodents, and people are severely punished for trying to exercise their freedoms of speech or religion.

Of course, in our own country, there are also serious, traumatic events. In our own country, children witness and experience domestic abuse every day. People are raped and brutally abused and murdered. People in the United States are homeless and hungry and live in deplorable conditions.

These things are tragic. But for those of us fortunate not to be suffering such trauma, I want to point out that we create the majority of our own misery. If you and your loved ones are relatively healthy, have gainful employment and can provide for your family (even if money is tight), if you have a roof over your head and food on your table (even if your roof leaks and your grocery budget is limited), you have the essential ingredients for contentment. If you are discontent with your life, then ask yourself, "What keeps me from being content in my life?" Chances are the answer is, in one way or another, related to your attitude and your thoughts about your circumstances, including your weight.

Response-ability

The author Stephen Covey notes that the word "responsibility" is the combination of the words "response" and "ability." Being responsible assumes being accountable. Responsible people are accountable for the choices they make. Ability implies competence. Response plus ability equals being accountable for using your competencies when making choices. Your own sense of contentment is within your control. You are able to achieve contentment. You are responsible for your own contentment. Again I ask: What stands in the way of your contentment/ happiness? What are you doing to pursue your own happiness/ contentment?

My favorite self-help author, John Friel, has discussed the difference between child-like thinking and adult-like thinking. Consider the following chart:

Child Thinking	Adult Thinking
I'm trapped.	I'm accountable.
I wait for others to make my life better.	I have choices.
I wait for others to change.	I find appropriate ways to meet my needs.
I wait for others to give me what I deserve.	I take charge of what needs to happen.

When we are caught up in addiction or negativity, we are stuck in child-like thinking. As an obese person, how often have you felt trapped? Feeling trapped may have been verbalized as "There's nothing I can do" or "I've tried everything and nothing works." As an obese person, have you waited for others to make your life better? Perhaps you expect people to wait on you in your home because you are too uncomfortable to do things yourself. Maybe you think it is your spouse's job or your child's job to make you happy? As an obese person, do you wait for others to change? Have you said things like, "If my husband would get help for his anger problem, I'd be happier and then I could lose weight?" Have you thought, "If my family would stop bringing junk food in the house, I wouldn't be surrounded by tempting food, and I could lose weight."? As an obese person, do you wait for others to give you what you deserve? Do you think, "I deserve a raise. If I got a raise, I'd be a happier person."? Have you complained, "People treat obese people badly. I deserve to be treated better by others. I'd be a more pleasant person if people were nicer to me."?

Adult thinking would go like this: "I'm not trapped by my obesity. The time has come for me to take responsibility for my health. I am accountable for making the changes in my eating and exercise habits, and I choose to begin today. I have choices as to how I want to go about losing weight. I can select a variety of food programs and I have numerous exercise options. I need to find ways to meet my own needs. I will seek counseling, whether or not my husband is willing to join me. I am joining the gym and will invite my family to go with me, but I'll go either way. I could opt to stay obese. If I do, I can't blame anyone else."

Obesity and Response-ability

Let's look at the idea of "response abilities" more closely. If you are obese, and if you do not want to remain obese, you are *responsible* and *able* to make the changes in your life that will result in your no longer being obese. Having bariatric surgery is a positive step. It is a responsible choice toward achieving your goal of better health and increased satisfaction with life. As you know, the surgery is only a tool to help you in the process of losing weight and keeping it off. You are responsible for, and able to, complete the Gotta Do Ems that are essential for sustained weight loss.

Contentment Response-ability

Choosing to make your life happier, more content, and more balanced in several arenas results in helping to balance your Enterprise Center. To attain this balance, you must take personal responsibility for the following:

- Choose to address your family history and work on issues that have contributed to your obesity and imbalance in your Enterprise Center.
- Choose to make your spiritual life the center of your world in order that you can find balance in your Enterprise Center.
- Choose what messages you were given about yourself that you want to keep and which you want to change; then get help in learning to change them.
- Choose what parenting techniques you learned from your parents that you want to keep and which you want to change; then get help in learning healthy parenting techniques.
- Choose what communication techniques you have learned that you want to get rid of (sarcasm, criticism) and get help in learning effective communication tools.
- Choose to set healthy boundaries with others; get help in learning how to set boundaries.
- Choose to set realistic, measurable goals and find ways to meet them, asking for help.

- Choose to implement physical activity and exercise into your life; then do it!
- Choose to learn and utilize positive thinking in your life and practice it daily.
- Choose to focus on gratitude in your life.
- Choose to have a healthy and balanced social life.
- Choose to work diligently to maintain balance in each of your Centers of Balance.
- Choose to complete the Gotta Do Ems daily!

A balanced Enterprise Center requires you to take personal responsibility for your choices and behaviors, especially your choices and behaviors related to eating and physical activity. Regardless of what happened in your childhood, regardless of what your current circumstances are, if you want to lose weight and keep it off, you are responsible for, and able to, engage in the behaviors necessary to do so.

Losing weight and keeping it off does not "just happen." No one can do the work it takes for you. Commitment and perseverance are necessary. Commitment and perseverance are choices you must make on a daily basis. William, who lives contentedly at 197 pounds after having surgery, said, "Sometimes I need to renew my commitment to my health on an hourly basis." He is right. Each time you are faced with an obstacle that threatens your weight loss, you must choose again to renew your commitment and to persevere.

As you gain a new sense of self by continuing to make choices that lead toward healthy living, you may also discover that you are able to make choices that bring your Enterprise Center back into balance. With the power gained from making healthy choices and implementing the thought processes and behaviors necessary to lose weight and keep it off, you may find that you are able to pursue the dreams and aspirations you thought impossible as an obese person.

Making these choices and staying true to them is a tough road, one that comparatively few people are able to follow. The final chapter of this book invites you to walk that road – the road too infrequently chosen.

Chapter 7: End of Chapter Exercises

Balance Brainwork

    1) Review your reasons for having weight loss surgery.

        a. What are five things you want to be different in your life as a result of having weight loss surgery?

        b. Write three to five specific steps to take to achieve each of the changes you noted above.

    2) Fill in the blank. "In order to give back to my community, I would like to find out more information on the following organizations, clubs or community events: _____

_____."

    3) Write a page on the following topic, which Steven Covey suggests, "How I want a) my children, b) my spouse, c) a co-worker, and d) a friend to describe me after I leave this world is:

_____."

    4) At the end of every day, ask yourself, "Today - have I lived up to the description of how I want others to describe me?"

Balance Busters

For each of the negative thought statements that follow, write down a positive statement to replace it.

Negative statement: "I'm too busy to get involved in community activities."
Positive statement: _____

_____.

Negative statement: "I don't see how being active in an organization will make a difference in my weight loss."
Positive statement: _____

_____.

Negative statement: "It would take too long to make my dream job a reality."
Positive statement: _____

_____.

Negative statement: "I can't imagine how I could leave a positive impact on this world."
Positive statement: _____

_____.

Balance Boosters
My dream job is _____

_____.

I choose to:
- develop specific goals so I can make this dream a reality in terms of my career, or
- develop specific goals so I can translate my dream job to a hobby or community involvement.

Three specific goals I have to make this happen are:
1.

2.

3.

I plan to give back to my community in the following three ways:
1.

2.

3.

The Best of the Best

- "For a community to be whole and healthy, it must be based on people's love and concern for each other." --   Millard Fuller
- "Be not afraid of life. Believe that life is worth living and your belief will help create the fact." -- William James
- "The real voyage of discovery consists not in making new landscapes but in having new eyes." -- Marcel Proust
- "We cannot seek achievement for ourselves and forget about progress and prosperity for our community. Our ambitions must be broad enough to include the aspirations and needs of others, for their sakes and for our own." -- Cesar Chavez
- "There can be no vulnerability without risk; there can be no community without vulnerability; there can be no peace, and ultimately no life, without community." -- M. Scott Peck

Cardinal Convictions

Write three Cardinal Convictions you will make part of your daily self-talk designed to remind yourself that balancing your Enterprise Center is essential to your long-term goals of sustained weight loss. For example: "I will give back to my community in ways that I enjoy, which is beneficial to me and to others."

Chapter 8

The Road Infrequently Traveled

Which do you choose when someone asks, "Do you want the good news or the bad news first?" I am going to share the good news with you first. The good news (there's lots of it) includes:

- Bariatric surgery is a wonderful way to help you lose weight and is often the only way for a morbidly obese person to lose a significant amount of weight.
- Hundreds of thousands of people are making the choice to begin a new and healthy life by having bariatric surgery.
- The health of surgical weight loss patients can be greatly improved following surgery.
- If you have made the choice to have bariatric surgery:
  - You are choosing to lose weight.
  - You are choosing to improve your health.

If you are reading this book:

- You have learned a great deal about obesity and the complex psychology associated with being obese.
- You have learned that you have choices about your thoughts and behavior.
- You are familiar with the Gotta Do Ems.

163

- You are aware of the need for maintaining equilibrium in all of your Centers of Balance.

Centers of Balance and Sustained Weight Loss

The natural and logical consequence of completing the Gotta Do Ems on a daily basis is sustained weight loss and a full, healthy life. The difference between those who lose their weight following surgery and keep it off and those who lose weight following surgery but gain a lot of it back is that the former group does the things necessary to keep their weight off: they make consistently healthy food choices, they maintain portion control, they exercise regularly, they drink water throughout the day, they eat breakfast, they plan their meals and follow their plan, they keep food and exercise journals, they get plenty of sleep, they utilize a healthy support system and, if necessary, they participate in individual and/or group counseling. You recognize these items? Good! That means you've been paying close attention throughout the book and know your Gotta Do Ems for sustained weight loss!

The road infrequently traveled leads to sustained weight loss and balance in life. The less than good news is that this road is infrequently traveled because "it's hard." To stay on this road requires a consistent determination to maintain a positive attitude, the perseverance to complete the GDEs on a daily basis, the courage to reach out and ask for help from others, the willingness to look at potentially painful emotional issues underlying obesity and a commitment to be your best self, the authentic person God placed you on this earth to grow into – before other people and the world had a chance to interfere. The road infrequently traveled leads to wonderful places: a life with good physical and emotional health, balanced Centers, and to living Contentedly-Ever-After.

Diets Don't Work

I have yet to meet a person preparing for bariatric surgery who has not gone on (and off) innumerable diets. The results are uniformly the same. "I lost weight until I went off the diet. Then I gained back all of the weight I lost plus some." Newsflash: Diets don't work.

Diets don't "work" for the following reasons:

- The implied goal of a diet is to lose weight, but *the real goal is to keep the weight off*. Diets only address losing weight.

- Many diets require people to eat pre-packaged food specific to that diet, exist on a liquid diet, follow a prescribed menu for a certain number of weeks, or reduce or eliminate an entire category of food. These "diets" won't work unless you are willing to do one of two things: 1) continue to eat the pre-packaged diet food, exist on a liquid diet, follow a prescribed menu, or reduce or eliminate an entire category of food *for the rest of your life*, or 2) eat healthy, balanced meals consisting of real food and refrain from "picking up where you left off" before the diet *for the rest of your life.*
- The diet may rely on diet pills. As soon as you quit taking diet pills, if you don't make the lifestyle changes required to stay at a healthy weight, you will gain your weight back.
- The diet may require consuming a very low number of calories. Any diet that results in significant weight loss is essentially a very low calorie diet. Add up the calories of one day's worth of the pre-packed diet food or the liquid "meals" or the prescribed food plans. What you will discover is that the total caloric intake is most likely less than 1200 calories per day.

Diets don't work, but bariatric surgery is designed to keep you from overeating. That's good news. The bad (or difficult) news is that is the only thing the surgery does. Weight-loss surgery ultimately does one thing and one thing only: It reduces the physical size of your stomach with the purpose of limiting the amount of food you can eat at one time. Period. Let me say that again. The lap band, the gastric sleeve, the gastric bypass … these procedures do only a very few things, one of which is to reduce the size of your stomach so as to limit the amount of food you can put into your stomach at one time.

Weight-loss surgery:

- *does not* keep you from putting cookies, candy, potato chips, or any other junk food into your mouth
- *does not* increase your motivation to exercise
- *does not* prevent cravings for food
- *does not* keep you from driving your vehicle through drive-thru windows at fast food restaurants
- *does not* keep family members from bringing mountains of tempting desserts to family reunions

- *does not* stop the holidays and all the goodies associated with those holidays
- *does not* keep co-workers from filling the break room with donuts, nor does it prevent them from wanting to go to the buffet at lunchtime.

You get the point. Your weight loss procedure will do one thing. It will create for you a small pouch in order to limit the amount of food you can put into your stomach at one time.

Beware the False Sense of Security

Whether you are preparing for surgery, have just had your surgery, or are several months past your surgery, beware the false sense of security that can develop in the first year following surgery. You WILL lose weight after surgery, and it may seem like you barely have to do anything to get those results. This is scary to me because the relative ease with which people lose the weight in the early months following surgery is often in SPITE of the lack of effort people put into it. This sets them up to think they can get away with not doing the things they need to do over the long haul to keep the weight off. People lose weight fairly easily during the first few months after the surgery because they are eating very little and don't want to physically harm their bodies as they adjust to their post-surgery body. Bariatric surgery patients are also usually very motivated immediately following the surgery, so they engage in healthy behaviors and start exercising.

These factors result in immediate weight loss, but this situation will not last. This initial period sets you up to think you can get away with not doing the things you need to do over the long haul to keep the weight off. Don't allow yourself to believe that you will continue to lose weight or that you will keep it off if you don't do a lot of things to keep it off. That is the false sense of security I refer to. You WILL have to do certain things to keep your weight off even if at first it seems like it just falls off!

I rarely have concerns about people losing their excess weight after surgery. Most do. I have tremendous concern about people not realizing that they can put their weight back on following the surgery. And many people do put their weight back on. People who gain their weight back often say things like, "The surgery didn't work." I remind them that the surgery doesn't work! It does nothing but keep them from putting too much food into their stomach at one time. *They* either work or *they* don't. You will have to work at making healthy food choices and you need to work at exercising on a regular basis. The surgery isn't intended to do any sort of "work." The patient is supposed to do the work.

Once you have lost your weight, you are at ground zero with all people who want to maintain their weight. When you attain a healthy weight at which you want to remain, you must maintain the behaviors that helped you lose the weight.

The surgical weight loss patients who regain all or a significant amount of their excess weight consume more calories than they burn. They do this by eating too much of the wrong foods too often. A lack of exercise, consistent grazing, and eating excessive amounts of simple carbohydrates found in "white foods" (foods made from white flour or sugar) and drinking alcohol ultimately result in unwanted pounds.

Yo-Yo Dieting and Weight Regain

Yo-Yo dieters "go on" diets and then "go off" diets. Logic dictates that "going off" a diet assumes a return to pre-diet behavior. Pre-diet behavior for an obese person involves eating too much of the wrong things too often. What would a person expect when they return to pre-diet behavior if not pre-diet weight?

Another of my favorite AA sayings is, "If you always do what you always did, you'll always get what you always got." In other words, if you were obese because you ate too much and didn't exercise before your surgery, you will be obese if you return to overeating and not exercising after your surgery.

The same holds true for people who have bariatric surgery. You must continue to eat healthy foods in reasonable portions and exercise regularly to maintain your weight loss. Regaining a large percentage of weight following bariatric surgery reduces the procedure to an enormously expensive and invasive diet.

Gotta Do Ems Along the Road

Let's review the Gotta Do Ems for Sustained Weight Loss Success one at a time. Make up your mind as you read about each that you are going to take the Road Infrequently Traveled. By doing so, you'll be one of the people who get the Results Too-Infrequently Obtained: sustained weight loss, improved health, and balanced Centers.

The Gotta Do Ems for Sustained Weight Loss Success
1) Make consistently healthy food choices (protein first)

When you have had weight loss surgery, your food choices become extremely important. The size of your pouch is approximately the size of an egg. Think about how much food you could fit into an egg shell. It's not much! Think about how much food you used to consume in one meal at a buffet… frightening! It's no wonder you lose weight quickly after surgery.

As I was writing this chapter, my mother shared with me an article from USA *Today*. The article reported that Denny's restaurant gave out free Denny's Grand Slam breakfasts for a period of eight hours. They fed 2 million people a meal consisting of two eggs, two slices of bacon, two sausage links, and two pancakes. Here are the nutrition facts from that Denny's Grand Slam breakfast:

Calories		760	
	Calories from fat	420	
			% daily value
Total fat		47 g	72%
	Saturated fat	14 g	70%
	Trans fat	0 g	
Cholesterol		475 mg	158%
Sodium		1,750 mg	73%
Total carbohydrate		57 g	158%
	Dietary fiber	3 g	73%
	Sugars	11 g	19%
Protein		28 g	12%

NOTE: This nutritional information does NOT include any butter, sugar, or other condiments added by the customer. (There are 100 calories in a tablespoon of butter, and approximately 110 calories in two tablespoons of maple syrup.)

Think about this! With butter and syrup, each of those 2 million people consumed approximately 1,000 calories in that one meal! ONE MEAL! You'll probably be eating about that many calories in an entire day after your surgery. And you'll need at least twice as much protein and a lot less fat in your 1,000 calories than are in a Denny's Grand Slam breakfast.

Your body, after surgery, will obtain all of its nutrition from the food you put into your egg-sized pouch three to five times a day. Because that small amount of food needs to provide your body with all of the nutrients it needs to remain healthy, your food choices need to be made exceptionally carefully. Your body needs up to 60 grams of protein every day after you have had a bariatric procedure. That's a lot of protein! And if you want the rewards of taking that Road Infrequently Traveled, you need to eat this way every single day.

You can get that protein from foods such as these:

Food	Quantity	Protein Grams
Egg	1 medium	6
Milk (skim)	1 cup	8
Soy milk	1 cup	6 - 10
Cottage Cheese (2%)	½ cup	16
Cheddar Cheese	1 ounce	7
Mozzarella, part skim	1 ounce	8
Ricotta cheese, part skim	½ cup	10
Yogurt, low-fat plain	1 cup	12
Roast chicken	4 ounces	31
Ground beef, extra lean	4 ounces	33

Food	Quantity	Protein Grams
Sirloin steak, choice cut, trimmed	4 ounces	35
Tuna, canned in water	4 ounces	33
Most fish fillets	3.5 ounces	22
Turkey breast, roasted no skin	4 ounces	24
Roast beef	3.5 ounces	28
Pork loin or tenderloin	4 ounces	29
Bacon	1 slice	3
Ham	3.5 ounces	18
Oatmeal	1 cup cooked	6
Rice, brown	1 cup cooked	5
Spaghetti	1 cup cooked	6
Whole wheat bread	2 slices	6
Almonds	1 ounce	6
Cashews, dry roasted	1 ounce	4
Peanuts	¼ cup	9
Pecans	¼ cup	2.5
Sunflower seeds	¼ cup	6
Flax seeds	¼ cup	8
Lentils	½ cup cooked	8
Lima beans	½ cup cooked	8
Peanut butter	2 Tbsp	10
Red kidney beans	½ cup canned	8
Soybeans	½ cup cooked	10
Tofu	4 ounces	9

You can add protein to your diet by consuming high quality protein bars (the more nutritious ones have at least 20 grams of protein per bar and have few fat grams) and protein shakes. You can enhance the flavor of the shakes by mixing them in the blender with ice and a tablespoon or two of sugar-free, fat-free whipped topping.

2) Maintain portion control

It's possible to consume too many calories of healthy food, which will eventually lead to weight regain. You may believe that because you had surgery, you won't be able to eat oversized portions. Initially, you won't be able to consume very much food at one time. But as your stomach relaxes, you will be able to eat more. Remain diligent about maintaining small portions!

One way post-surgical patients lose control of portion size is by grazing. Grazing is grazing, regardless of whether the food you put in your mouth is healthy or not. Grazing amounts to eating too much. Eating too much results in gaining weight. It's important to eat at regular intervals so you keep track of when and how much you eat. When you graze or eat mindlessly, as when eating while watching television or reading, you aren't aware of how much food you consume. Even though your stomach pouch is the size of an egg, if you fill it continually all day long, you will consume a lot of food and a lot of calories over the course of a day. Eat your meals at prescribed times and be aware of making healthy food choices in sensible portions.

Your surgeon and nutritionist gave you instructions on what and how to eat. I can confidently say that no health care professional has instructed you, or has given you permission to eat large portions of food, to graze, or to eat unhealthy foods.

3) Exercise daily

Talk about a road infrequently traveled. Rare is the person who exercises daily. Extremely rare is the person who exercises daily consistently over time throughout their adult lives. Extraordinarily rare is the Yo-Yo dieter who remains diligent about exercising on a daily basis for an extended period of time. To sustain your weight loss you must exercise on a consistent basis. No exceptions. No excuses. Read Chapter 4 whenever you are tempted to skip exercise!

4) Drink plenty of water throughout the day, but not with meals

There are several reasons your surgeon and nutritionist tell you to refrain from drinking liquids at mealtime. When you drink liquids, you fill your pouch with fluid. Drinking water is a well-known "diet tip" to help people feel full. Because your pouch is so small, and you need to get optimal nutrition from healthy food at meal time, you don't want your pouch to be filled with liquid. If half of your egg-sized pouch is full of water before you eat, you may not feel hungry at meal time and therefore you may not eat enough to get sufficient nutrition.

You don't want to drink fluids during the course of your meal because doing so may allow you to eat more than you need to. Drinking can force food to be pushed through from your pouch more quickly than it should be, allowing room for more food. The more food you consume, the more calories you consume. And as you know, the more calories you consume, the greater your weight will be.

You certainly don't want to drink fluids after you eat a complete meal, either. Drinking after your pouch is already filled with food leads to the excess being expelled... that's right, you vomit.

5) Eat breakfast

What's the big deal about eating breakfast? According to MayoClinic. com, "A healthy breakfast refuels your body and replenishes your blood sugar (glucose), giving you the energy necessary to start a new day. In addition, a growing body of evidence indicates that breakfast is good for both your physical and mental health." Breakfast is also important as it wakes your metabolism up after it, like you, has been sleeping during the night. You want to lose weight and keep it off, so get your metabolism running first thing in the morning. Eating breakfast also keeps you from getting so hungry later in the day that you are more likely to overeat when you finally put food into your system. It has also been noted that eating breakfast increases your concentration and improves your thinking, leads to eating more nutritionally throughout the day, and increases energy.

6) Plan your meals and follow your plan.

I hear you groaning. I know... I know... it's hard, you don't have time, it takes a lot of effort, blah, blah, blah. When you went on various other diets, you planned meals. The problem was, when you "went off" the diet, you stopped planning your meals, and you stopped following your plan. Do it again, only this time, keep following your food plan. For life – one day at a time. One of my favorite mottos is, "Work smarter, not harder." In this case, those words translate to keeping your food plans on your computer. Once you have fifteen or twenty days of meals planned, you can mix and match. That doesn't take much time!

Be sure when you plan your meals that you take into consideration your work schedule, your kids' extracurricular activities and other issues that make eating on a routine schedule difficult. It may be that a protein bar is a meal if you are on the go. A can of low fat soup high in protein is a quick meal you can heat up at the office. Small cans of tuna or chicken salad with whole wheat crackers makes for a nice lunch as does instant oatmeal and a hard-boiled egg white. Work smarter – not harder.

Making your meal plans won't be as difficult as following them. You will have to utilize your new skill of setting healthy boundaries when it comes to eating right. Your friends at the office will have to understand that you are bringing your lunch and won't be joining them every day at a restaurant. The kids will need to get used to the fact that you don't keep junk food in the house. Your mother-in-law can choose to have her feelings hurt or not when you tell her not to bring baked goods to your house. Your health and your life depend on following your food plan.

7) Keep food and exercise journals

This sounds like two different tasks. However, you would be wise to keep one journal where you record your food and exercise for the day. (It's that smarter not harder concept again.) However, some people have found food or exercise diaries online they are partial to. It doesn't matter how you choose to journal. It matters *that* you choose to journal.

I can't emphasize just how important this is. There are so many reasons for you to record both what you eat and the amount of time and kind of exercise that you do. Maintaining food and exercise journals provides a measure of accountability.

As noted in Chapter 5, people underestimate how much they eat by 20% and more. Writing down every bite of food that goes in your mouth prevents you from lying to yourself about what you have actually eaten.

Keeping a food diary may be *the most* beneficial tool you can use to maintain your weight loss. If you start gaining weight, you can look back in your journal and see what you are doing differently. If you are gaining weight, you are either eating more, exercising less, or a combination of the two. When people say, "My weight just crept back on," they are not being accountable for their behavior. Weight is gained by overeating and/or not exercising.

Keeping food and exercise journals doesn't have to be a huge ordeal. Most cell phones have a "notes" section on them. Jot down what you eat at the time you eat it. That way you don't have to try to recount the entire day's food intake later (which leads to inaccuracy of recall). At the end of the day, whether you use an online diary or have a spiral notebook at home, you can simply transfer the information from your cell phone to your journal.

Remember the importance of keeping your thoughts positive. When it comes to maintaining food and exercise journals, tell yourself, "I don't really want to do this, but if I don't, I may not lose the weight I want to, and it will be difficult to keep it off. Therefore, I choose to write down what I eat and my exercise for the day. This is a top priority in my life this day and every day." Once you have claimed journaling as a part of what you do each day, there is no longer any debate about whether or not you have time, or if you feel like it or not. You have made it a priority and you do it!

Keeping food and exercise journals helps you recognize and solve problems. If you discover that you do very well during the day but overeat in the evening, you can figure out what you will do to correct that problem.

Your journals will also help strengthen your motivation. Take time each week and each month to review your eating behaviors. Give yourself credit for developing and maintaining healthy habits and for sticking to your plan. This, in turn, helps you build confidence. Seeing success increases your desire to continue succeeding.

Do yourself a huge favor. ACCEPT that you must choose to write down what you eat and how you exercise each day. It's a good idea to make yourself keep a weight graph, too. A graph is a great visual reminder that you are losing weight. When you reach the weight your body settles into, maintain the graph over time. If the line on the graph starts to rise, indicating an increase in your weight, it means you are doing something differently. The goal is to keep your excess weight off. If you are regaining, review your food and exercise journals, discover where the problems lie, make a plan to "get back to the basics" (meaning doing what you did to lose the weight in the first place) and implement your plan.

8) Get plenty of sleep

"Chronic sleep deprivation may cause weight gain by affecting the way our bodies process and store carbohydrates, and by altering levels of hormones that affect our appetite," reported in the January 2006 edition of *Harvard Women's Health Watch*.

Getting enough sleep is a challenge for most of us. We have busy lives, and sleep seems to be one of the first things we give up. Do yourself and the rest of the family a favor and make getting enough sleep a priority for all of you. Besides keeping your weight steady, getting enough sleep will prevent you from being grumpy, will keep your thinking sharper, and will protect your overall health.

9) Utilize a healthy support system (support group meetings and online support)

No one can do the work of weight loss for you; yet, you can't do it alone. You are the one who has to make the choice to lose weight and follow through with each of the Gotta Do Ems. Your spouse can't be responsible for what you put in your mouth. Your children can't be responsible for whether or not you exercise. Your friends can't make you keep a food and exercise journal. Only you can do these things.

But you can't do it alone. You need encouragement, which your spouse, children, and friends can give you. You need education, which your doctor and nutritionist can give you. You need knowledge that comes from experience, which others who have been through the process can give you.

Attend the local support group meetings for bariatric patients. Befriend others who truly understand the process you are going through. Assist others as they begin their journeys. Join online groups for people who have had weight loss surgery. Many have 24-hour forums where you can post questions and get feedback from peers and professionals. Remember: "You can't keep it if you don't give it away."

10) Participate in individual and/or group counseling for at least a year

Those of you who are the most serious about keeping your weight off will pick up the phone and make an appointment with a qualified therapist right now, if you haven't been attending therapy already. Those of you who think you don't need this are fooling yourselves. Can you lose weight without attending therapy? Of course! Can you keep your weight off without attending therapy?

Perhaps, but I have seen and heard with my eyes and ears the stories of people just like you (and don't forget, I am a recovering addict). I know about the issues underlying addiction, and how hard they are to change. I have been to therapy myself. I know firsthand the benefits of having a professional help you work through the issues underneath your "problem."

Weight loss following bariatric surgery is about learning to live life on life's terms; learning to deal with your thoughts and feelings without using food to alleviate sadness, pain, anger, loneliness, or boredom. Work with your therapist to break your bad eating habits and learn new, healthy habits. Let a professional teach you how to recognize negative, sabotaging thoughts, and replace them with helpful ways of thinking and behaving. Losing weight is difficult. Keeping it off, even more so. Give yourself a gift and get into therapy. You'll be amazed at how much better you feel every time you leave a session (even if you leave in tears)! You will also have balance in each and every one of your Centers much sooner than someone not attending therapy.

The Goals

As you finish this book, my hope for you is that your goals following weight loss surgery include:

- Losing your excess weight
- KEEPING THE EXCESS WEIGHT OFF FOR A LIFETIME
- Improving your overall health
- Living a full, balanced life in your Spiritual Center, your Cognitive Center, your Emotional Center, your Physical Center, your Social Center, and your Enterprise Center

In addition to giving my patients a chart with the Gotta Do Ems, I give them a green silicone bracelet to wear that reads: "MY HEALTH, MY RESPONSIBIITY... THIS DAY. EVERY DAY." It might sound trite, but living one day at a time is a great way to live. Staying in the day, not worrying about tomorrow, next week or next year, has saved many a recovering alcohol a trip down hangover lane. It can save you a trip there yourself, whether it be a hangover from alcohol, too much food, or from a night of self-pity and anger.

Samantha, three years post-surgery, minus 125 pounds, and doing exceptionally well in her life, told me, "I hated that 'one day at a time' idea before I figured out what a gift it is for me! I struggled a lot my first year after surgery. I was grieving the loss of my favorite sugary foods. I was sad and angry thinking about how I could NEVER have another piece of chocolate cake again in my life. But my therapist helped me realize it was my choice to NOT eat chocolate cake or candy bars. It relieved me to know that tomorrow I might have chocolate cake or candy or ice cream, but 'today,' whatever day it was, I was choosing not to. I felt at peace and I felt empowered. For the most part, I am doing well now, staying away from too much sugar, living life more fully and making healthy food choices one day at a time."

Just for today, make a conscious decision to:
- make consistently healthy food choices (protein first)
- maintain portion control
- exercise daily
- drink plenty of water throughout the day, but not with meals
- eat breakfast
- plan your meals and follow your plan
- keep food and exercise journals
- get plenty of sleep
- utilize a healthy support system (support group meetings and on-line support)

Gratefully Yours

You have taken a lot of time to read these pages, and I hope you have learned some things about what you need in the years ahead to keep your weight off - one day at a time.

I wrote this book as much for myself as for you. I know the importance of sharing what I have learned along my journey in recovery. Not much that comes out of my mouth or my mind is original, but my way of passing it on has originality. So many people have blessed my life, sharing their wisdom, strength, experiences and sometimes a swift kick to my rear. Hopefully, by sharing these words, you will take from them what you need. I will remember that, like you, I am responsible for the effort I put into whatever I do.

Your health is, after all, your responsibility. This day. Every day.

With gratitude to you, I close this chapter and this book, leaving with you the theme of my life's work through a quote from George Herbert (1593-1633): "Give Thanks. Thou who has given us so much. Mercifully grant us one more thing— a grateful heart."

For gratitude, I believe, is the key to happiness.